A 50-Year **YOGA SOMATIC** Journey
From Chaos to Calm

REACH

and

RECEIVE

Diana Devi

*The strategies and advice presented in this
book are not a substitute for medical advice
or professional counseling. Seek guidance from
qualified professionals for personalized support.*

patients and with our formerly over-scheduled, busy, mentally and physically stressed yoga group who were then guided so gently through the pandemic by her online Zoom classes but most importantly, by her whole yoga-centric philosophy of life."

—NEIL JOHNSON, MD

"Diana's fifty-year transformational journey is a testament to the power and impact of yoga practice in helping us break through the mental, emotional, and physical barriers to our success, health, and happiness. Because our individual growth and evolution affect the whole of humanity, it is more important than ever to awaken to a new way of being as we navigate these challenging and troubling times. Reach and Receive *is an inspirational must-read for anyone ready to activate their personal power and create heaven on earth."*

—KEIYA K. RAYNE, CEO, SOUL STRATEGY
COACHING, AND TEDx SPEAKER

"Reaching out to the universe every morning to receive its gifts is already an injection of progress. Whether you need to heal from illness or loss, Diana's book, Reach and Receive, *immediately draws you into a critical reminder that we have vast tools to tap into for our wellbeing and growth. She doesn't spare details when using her own life as an instrument of change. You'll come to know this inspirational figure while learning new poses and breathwork from a master!"*

—DONNA SIRLIN, AUTHOR OF HEALING THROUGH
HAPPINESS, AND WELLNESS INFLUENCER

"Authentic and heart-centered, Diana Guy will sweep you into her storytelling, making you feel right there with her on her yoga journey (minus the sweat). Her account, from chaos to calm, will inspire you to want to start yoga right now. She built the plane while flying and has shown us that even when you're afraid, anything is possible when you trust your inner guidance system and surrender to the process, knowing you will be supported and shown the way."

—SHARON HOLAND GELFAND, INTEGRATIVE NUTRITIONIST AND TRANSFORMATION COACH, SPEAKER AND AUTHOR OF *THE G.U.T. METHOD*

"Diana Guy is an intrepid somatic explorer, who knows how to follow somatic intuition, how to go beneath and beyond the common experiences and descriptions of a body, and sensuously experience the primordial and cosmic dimensions of emergent life. In the early 80s, Diana sponsored me to bring Continuum workshops to Cincinnati, where I witnessed her enthusiastically opening into novel sensuous life-changing experiences. She understood the ramifications of such experiences as they unfolded into every aspect of living an embodied creative life. Out of all her years of teaching and diving into the mysteries, Diana has written this delicious memoir with a heart wish to spark your curiosity and value for your own unfolding journey. It includes a practice guide designed to help you create a practice that inspires vibrant health and well-being, and a deep unfolding of your unique sacred heart."

—SUSAN HARPER, MSME/T, CONTINUUM TEACHER AND DEVELOPER OF BODY OF RELATING, PORTALS OF PERCEPTION, AND LIVING DREAMS SEMINARS

"Reach and Receive *offers readers a journey from chaos to calm, reducing stress by encouraging the creation of moments to pause and focus attention. Finding time to connect with nature and reduce the noise of day-to-day commitments is at the heart of promoting health and well-being.*"

—CINDY WILLCOCKS, QN, DIRECTOR AND
REGISTERED MENTAL HEALTH NURSE

"Reach and Receive *is an amazing self-revelatory story of her journey from chaos to calm. Diana chronicles her life's path with vulnerability and honesty. I took my first yoga class from Diana in the 90s, and she was an awesome teacher. In order to wake up from ordinary consciousness, three things are required: a Buddha, Sanga, Dharma. Diana helps us understand the path to 'awakening' via her journey with all three keys: Lilias, the teachings, and her community. This is a must read for anyone on the journey of awakening. This is a story of the student who becomes a master.*"

—DEBORAH OOTEN, PH.D., CEO/OWNER, CONSCIOUS
LIVING CENTER AND CONSCIOUS DYNAMICS, LLC

"*Since the early 1990s, when Diana began teaching at the Cancer Support Community (formerly The Wellness Community), she has provided stress relief and balance to thousands affected by cancer. In the challenging landscape of cancer treatment, Diana serves as a beacon of hope, extending her role beyond conventional yoga instruction to become a source of strength and solace for those navigating the emotional and physical distress of cancer. Diana's remarkable dedication is evident in her tailored yoga sessions, addressing the unique needs of cancer patients facing physical limitations and emotional hurdles. Her adaptive approach recognizes the distinct journey of each individual, fostering inclusivity and empowerment.*

Beyond physical benefits, Diana cultivates a supportive community within her classes, countering the isolating nature of cancer with camaraderie. This sense of belonging significantly contributes to the emotional healing process, providing a safe space for expression without judgment."

—KELLY SCHOEN (SHE/HERS), EXECUTIVE DIRECTOR, CANCER SUPPORT COMMUNITY GREATER CINCINNATI-NORTHERN KENTUCKY

"Diana Guy's book is a thorough romp through the yoga world of self-discovery. You will be introduced to the luminaries as her personal history unfolds along with many of the friends she met along the way. It's high spirited and oh, so much fun. The book shows that to get to calm there is a journey and you have to participate. Jump in, see where you land."

—JEAN COUCH, AUTHOR, *THE RUNNER'S YOGA BOOK*, AND SENIOR TEACHER OF BALANCE, THE WORK OF NOELLE PEREZ

Table of Contents

Acknowledgments

It takes a village....

Family, friends, peers, and participants are truly so many, my Acknowledgments could be a lovely short story.

I am grateful for Candi Cross, my persistent and passionate editor and dear friend, who has nudged me for many years to write my story of yoga and included me in a few of her clients' books as reference. She is responsible for seeing this project finally manifest to the finish line.

Kathy Simes, graphic designer extraordinaire, created a cover both personal and beautiful and who also edited all photos. Her work was invaluable and professional, and her availability was so appreciated! Cousin love!

Evan Noyes, my IT specialist answered the call ("Help Evan, I can't figure out this system!"), saved the manuscript and was always amazing and available with his IT knowledge. Love my grandson bunches!

Vickie Fairchild, yoga teacher, physical therapist and author of *Divine Trilogy* for saying "Yes!" to model the yoga asanas for a necessary visual cueing for readers. A friendship of lifetimes with adventures in living our best life!

Teachers/mentors inspiring and lifting me up during my journey include these remarkable beings: Lilias Folan, Emilie Conrad,

Rev. Carol Parrish, Sita Frenkel, Swami Chidananda, Swami Pranananda, Robert Fulford, MD, Jack Armstrong, DC, Jean Couch, Susan Harper, Sister Mary Alexander, RSM, Sister Julie, SND. CYTA teachers and friends, Jerrilee Lucas, Jan Kolish, Jill McConnell, Kathy Hunter, Roger Null, Nancy Bloemer. Oh, so many more past, present, and future! You all inspire me!

Kathryn Jones, BodyMindMovement, San Francisco, sharing our love of Continuum and inspiring each other always in all ways in our work and a forever friendship.

Those who honored my work and shared with cover stories and awards and teaching opportunities throughout the years, I am grateful! Especially Suzie Collins of *New Lifestyle Magazine* and Atif Kemaz of WorldBeat Productions. The TV and radio programs/interviews on local Cincinnati stations and other cities were fun and a stimulating source in my journey! Kelly Schoen for submitting me for an Unsung Hero Award for Cancer Family Care.

Jenny Bird, musician-singer in the 70s singing in my classes, retreats and taking me to the Land of Enchantment New Mexico for healing. This sparked my journey with my first radio interview, living simply and valuing energy of sacred mountain and land. Spiritual resonance and friend for life!

Jeanette Wiesner, RN, TriHealth, P&G, Lynn Stern, The Wellness Community now Cancer Support Community, Jesuit community for local and international retreat opportunities. Many organizations and individuals who sponsored me nationally and internationally. I am honored and deeply grateful!

First readers who said "Yes!" with no hesitation and waited for months as I crawled to my finish line/finished lines: Jean Couch, Sharon Holand Gelfand, Susan Harper, Amy Henry, Neil Johnson,

MD, Deborah Ooten, Ph.D., Keiya Rayne, Kelly Schoen, MSW, Donna Sirlin, and Cindy Willcocks, QN. Your feedback/endorsements had me in tears!

Yoga participants in classes, retreats, private sessions, workshops, you always inspire a deeper dive and curiosity! Your continued support of my journey is a valued expression of love and your unique journey. I am so grateful! My Tuesday morning students, P&G retirees and weekly Zoomers, love you all! Also, over thirty years sharing with cancer patients, you all touch me with your accessing of somatic realms for healing and heartfelt courage during vulnerable moments.

Sadie, my dear yogi dog who missed walks, treats, ball-chasing moments for this book, and always shows up on my yoga mat demonstrating the value of stretching, dog pose especially, physical patting, and unconditional love for self and another.

My amazing kids, Angie, Jamie, and Brad, who grew up with a yogi mom and who matured with an integrity and empathy and are amazing parents of my extraordinary grandkids! You are and always have been an integral part of my journey. My love for you three beautiful gifts in my life is immeasurable! Rice cakes, crystals and all the moments you endured—oh my! Mike, Sue and Piradee, thank you for being in our family and supportive of all we do.

Grandkids Sara, Riley, Abby, Julianne, Evan, Sidney, Ryan, Ella, and Ethan, you all make me strive to be a better person and to deeply love. My heart of hearts!

My sister, Mary, an incredible example of surviving cancer, for creating beautiful bookmarks for my book. You are the crafty one, to be sure! Your support and kindness are precious.

My cousins, Barbie and Marian, for a memorable East Coast beach trip and sunrise beach yoga photos (including the cover photo of this book).

Finally, YOU, the reader, I am grateful you picked up my book and hope you are inspired in some way to be enthused, be curious and find what sparks your exciting journey this lifetime.

YES, YOU CAN! Let's do this together!

Introduction

Zoom On into the Future of Yoga

> *"Try to find pleasure in the speed that you're not used to. Changing the way you do routine things allows a new person to grow inside of you. But when all is said and done, you're the one who must decide how you handle it."*
>
> —Paulo Coelho

WALKING OUT OF P&G, where I've taught yoga and holistic work for over twenty-five years, into the breezy March air, I'm chilled by the early-spring temperature and the unknown virus spreading across the globe. Two longtime students, Jane and Susan, showed up braving the uncertainty of being in proximity with fellow practitioners while breathing in new life or spreading of a potential deadly contagion, COVID-19. They physically separated six feet apart in what will become our new norm for safe distancing. Jane and Susan were the only two who showed up for our usually filled class that day.

"Two weeks off," the desk supervisor stated to me on March 15, 2020, "until this 'thing' settles down."

Five months later, I'm setting up in my home for Zoom class. Lights, microphone, tutorials regarding navigation of site, an online workshop with a photographer regarding lighting and colors for nails and full appearance on screen. Gathering HDMI cords, positioning the TV screen and laptop in the correct height for camera angles to capture standing, lying down and sitting movements, all encompass a new avenue and challenges for teaching yoga. As I position all this and open the Zoom room twenty minutes before class, I am drawn back to my first moments fifty years ago, walking into a school gym to practice yoga for the first time.

Thousands of students, infinite hours traversing my teaching certifications, retreats and symposiums, classes for every type of population imaginable, all fashioning an illustrious journey, brings me from then to this moment in my home where I await a few dozen participants from different cities on the screen. This may be a pivotal moment—retire or return with IT skills and continue, just in a new way. My passion and enthusiasm for yoga always wins out with a vocation, which began in a school gym in September of 1973.

I can still smell the aroma of the gym wood floor, see the impactful room of people decked out in leotards and tights, the oversized, old windows we would open to allow fresh air if it was too warm, and the stage where Lilias, our teacher who amassed fame from her PBS series, "Lilias, Yoga and You", would position herself so she could see out over many rows of participants.

It was the 1970s, and with people emerging from the turbulent 60s, Jimmy Carter was elected President and initiated a program assisting low-income families to obtain a new home. That is how my then husband and I purchased and built a home in the suburbs. While lounging in the backyard with my children playing with neighborhoods kids on our swing set, I would be reading yoga books and writing intently in pencil about my awakening through yoga. The pages of my journal contained an outpouring of fear and excitement for life chapters that would expose, strengthen, and test me to my core during a critical reinvention.

I felt a tremendous surge of change trembling within my core and fear of the unknown. Where would and could this yoga possibly be carrying me? Me, a mother of three little ones, a typical 1970s housewife having this tidal wave of dynamic, creative change. A life reaching out from within the depths of my heart, a knowing there is a better way of being in love, good health with joy. With unmeasurable fear and excitement, this all began to unfold. The healing was initiated when I walked through the doors into my first yoga class. Healing from anxiety and depression, and from an immune deficiency I did not know existed until many years later. In this twenty-minute interval before Zoom class, I made rose tea to soothe my vocal cords. But due to extreme shyness and anxiety, I would have uttered only a few words in a crowd to begin with. There, she sat cross-legged on a mat on the stage, her dark, braided hair draped over her shoulder. Our eyes caught each other when I entered, and she smiled a most welcoming smile. In hindsight, we *recognized* each other from an ancient time. It had felt like returning *home* in that one moment. Her radiant smile formed as an acknowledgement of reunion, seeing each other.

Fifty years ago, wow! Forward bends, arches, spinal moves, and breathing exercises from then through now assist my own body in feeling flexible, stronger, energized and calmer. How blessed I am to have made it through the elementary school gym doors that September evening of 1973 against so many odds.

The whistling of the tea kettle signaled for me to return to the present. Another check of Zoom sound, lighting, and positioning of camera before strolling out onto my patio with Sadie, my rescue dog who always makes a cameo appearance in class and entertains the participants in more poses than the Downward Dog.

While outdoors, I paused by the water feature to meditate, listen, and absorb the early morning sounds of birds singing, water trickling, evening crickets fading out their conversations. This so soothes my body and centers me. Communing with nature—other beings in my garden including flowers, plants, chipmunks, bunnies, and squirrels—bonds me to an inclusive part of my ritual for awakening upon Mother Earth.

Sipping and stirring my senses, I wandered back to 1973, when we could not have imagined this morning's tech scenario, as one wall phone usually positioned in a kitchen was our way of remotely communicating with others. This kitchen, decorated in 70s Spanish-themed sconces in gold and green colors, would become a healing center to explore various dietary changes from sugar and meats to healthier choices with many benefits for me, my family and even our dog, Kali Shanti. Yoga and the uplifting community that ensued saved me, transformed me into something so magnificent—a divine magnificence that initiated a lifetime vocation of helping others transform their lives from chaos to calm. In this power, I would go on to pioneer healing programs for drug and alcohol residential rehab, cancer and other immune disorders, corporate health, prenatal and chair yoga, and somatic movement blends.

You will come to know this magnificence in its pure form is yours for the taking, too. It is your birthright to change, grow, flourish in unknown territory outside and within you!

As I finished preparing for my class, I told myself that I would call Lilias today to schedule another lunch date. We live fifteen minutes apart and have enjoyed a reunion this past year. The words, "I am blessed", filled my mind, heart, body as I arose from the serene patio and entered my Zoom session. I heard the participants chatting with so much vibrancy and gratitude to be alive and having an opportunity to connect with each other during this once-in-a-lifetime pandemic. What a joy they are, and this experience is, for me! "The joy is in the journey" is a topic Lilias coined and shared with many others.

With this journey of fifty years in yoga, I walk upon a path that is sometimes winding, sometimes steep, sometimes flat, sometimes soft, sometimes painful, and yes, joyful but always moving and unfolding into the greater awareness of who I am and my deepest connections upon this earth, this lifetime.

Oh, how the pandemic of COVID-19 has thrown all aspects of life up in the air including yoga teaching and studying. I summoned more resilience and resourcefulness to fulfill a need in students who were vulnerable from aging, cancer and other diseases, anxiety and stress disorders, dementia—while also staying employed and creating a new path of entrepreneurship from bottom up. I was up to the challenge.

Sadie and I walked into our Zoom room. I tuned into my Sacred Heart and higher self while connecting individually and collectively with those enthusiastic yogis appearing on my screen. I also paused to feel into those who could not be with us for whatever reason.

In this new digital way to be together, I am still inspired by each one attending. I get so excited to see and feel what may possibly unfold in our collective heart, mind, bodies this morning.

This is my story, my eclectic path. I hope you find a connection, a spark of curiosity and value for your own journey and share your story with someone today. Storytelling, as ancient as earth itself, is a vital tool for continuing on this earth. Our evolution unfolds with all species communicating and contributing.

The Practice Guide is designed to help you create a practice that inspires vibrant health and wellness, body-mind-spirit. And perhaps, a deep unfolding of your Sacred Heart into each new day! Beginners and teachers alike can benefit. I encourage you to read a section, put the book down and practice a few moments. The health benefits will soon appear for you.

Also, I am here for contact if you'd like a personal one-on-one consultation or instruction. I am always enthusiastic to mentor and to be of service in any way possible. Carrying on this lineage of teaching is within my heart of hearts on my journey.

I was honored to be mentored by the most incredible teachers in yoga, other movement modalities and spiritual awakening pathways. Their guidance and mentoring, even fifty years later, encourages and prompts me to continue to learn, to be curious in my unfolding into a greater life. My words can only be a snippet of their unique intelligence and generous love. I continue to feel them support my journey, appearing and nudging me in most curious ways and welcome the new adventures. They inspire me to carry on and evolve the story.

PART I

Flow And Tell:
The Fifty-Year Journey

Chapter 1

'Lilias, Yoga and You'...and Me

> *"Within ourselves, there are voices that provide us with all the answers that we need to heal our deepest wounds, to transcend our limitations, to overcome our obstacles or challenges, and to see where our soul is longing to go."*
>
> —DEBBIE FORD

September 1973

I JOINED FAMILY AND neighbors for a night out, away from young children and the daily grind of keeping our sanity and a sense of who we were before we became mothers, wives, and the chaos that was inherent in this culture.

"I signed us all up for yoga class with Lilias Folan, who is on TV!" shouted my cousin, Donna, from her wall phone and while puffing on a cigarette.

"YOGA?" I exclaimed with a painful, hoarse voice due to bronchitis, which infected my feverish body. I thought, *why not bowling or another artsy activity such as ceramics or watercolor painting?*

"She's on PBS TV, watch her tomorrow!" she continued with enthusiasm how much fun we would have on top of this privilege being taught by a TV star in our neighborhood adult education program.

It's not that I wasn't curious. I just couldn't feel all the perks of curiosity because illness and anxiety were overriding awe. At twenty-three, my body was feverish and achy, surviving through shallow breath and depression. Fatigue was a chronic life curse and with three little ones with high energy clamoring for attention, I felt at times, I was unable to keep the pace and the faith. A marriage in turmoil with stressful days and nights that were accumulating fears and anxieties was not the vision I formed of a happy-ever-after fairytale wedding and life. These three little, beautiful beings, who I birthed, were the constant motivation during a turbulent time. I thank God they were a part of my life and journey as they kept through chaos a stream of love and purpose.

The concept of yoga was foreign, completely estranged from my life and as a "night out". I vowed to check out this famous yoga lady and looked her up on the schedule in *Cincinnati Enquirer's* "TV Guide". Sure enough, there was the "Lilias, Yoga and You" show on PBS. I have an autographed copy of this guide with Lilias on their cover. This is one of many yoga artifacts I have in my possession.

The following morning, after the kids ate breakfast, dressed, and headed outdoor for adventurous neighborhood playing, I turned on the program to see what I was getting myself into (or getting myself out of). I recall sitting there, curled up on my couch with our furry family member, Brittany, the flexible calico cat. As the program began, I was mesmerized by her calming voice and radiant smile in an instant. Lilias's ability to seemingly make me feel like I was the only one she was focused upon in my living room was a gift she offered for thousands who tuned in each TV episode I would soon discover. Her long, dark brown, braided hair cascaded over her shoulder; her radiant smile and eyes, and gentle, caring voice welcomed me into the world of yoga. I did, indeed, get off my sofa as she suggested, onto my carpeted floor and began my first yoga practice in 1973.

Lilias would instruct me from her show for a month each day prior to our family night out. I was surprised by the simplicity of poses and instruction on TV, which enabled me to delicately enter my journey with yoga. I became very anxious to meet her and realized what a privilege it would be to be instructed by someone so known and respected.

Day of. My sisters, in-laws, their friends and my neighbor and I contacted each other with great anticipation for our upcoming class that eve. All I could think about was class and putting my moves to the test with a living being other than my cat, who soared past me in agility and flexibility every time. *What to wear, what to bring…* "loose fitting clothing, a towel or a non-slip rug". I do not recall the outfit, but my first mat was a powder blue bathmat with enough length to support my head and torso down to my tailbone. The non-slip rubber backing on the school gym floor was great too. It wasn't long before a few of us caravanned to a Capezio store to purchase a leotard (mine was bright yellow, which I kept as another yoga artifact) and a pair of black tights. We were instructed to cut out the bottom so we could put our bare feet through them for standing poses.

As my neighbor friend and I pulled up into the parking lot, which was filled with potential neophyte yogis carrying in an assortment of towels, rugs, I noticed we were of all sizes and ages as we stood in a long line to be signed in. Sixty-five participants crowded into the school gym. As I entered through the double wooden doors with great anticipation, there Lilias was sitting cross-legged up on the stage, smiling as we all filed through perhaps an invisible doorway into our new life and way of being. As I said in the intro, our eyes met. Her welcoming smile with "Namaste" gesture familiarized by her TV show initiated this relationship into a mentorship and friendship. This moment of our first "seeing" initiated a caring relationship which will unfold unto this present day, decades later, as we continue to share lunch and life stories. As Lilias spoke, I felt so grateful for her presence in my life.

My crew all quickly ran to the back of the room and lined up, creating our own row, giggling, and getting ready to do yoga for our night out. A virtual sea of yogi participants in front of us to the seeming faraway stage. Lilias's voice projected quite well to the back of the room as she welcomed us all and introduced her assistants, two women who sat beside her, and herself.

We sat upon our towels, bathmats, rugs, eagerly awaiting our instructions. After a warm address that included a brief on her own yoga history, she asked us to lie down in *Sarvasana*, introducing an ancient language. We were prompted to note how we felt throughout our body. The giggling persisted in our row and around the room, overlaying whispered comments. I recall what occurred that night and share with students to this day as an example of what some of them may be going through. At a very young age of twenty-three, my crazy mind was rambling short, half sentences with jumbled and disconnected thoughts though my body was still. *Am I insane?* I asked myself this question since I had not noticed the chaotic mind before. This was a eureka moment for me. Besides an inflexible body, my chaotic mind was also an impetus to start and continue with commitment to change my daily habits toward a healthier lifestyle. Without that moment of committing to a now vocation of yoga practice and teaching, I wonder where I would be, or even if I would be here today.

Harvard Medical School, along with other respectable institutions, got it right years later when they declared that yoga strengthens parts of the brain that play a key role in memory, attention, awareness, thought, and language, and can affect mood by elevating levels of a brain chemical called *gamma-aminobutyric acid* (GABA), which is associated with better mood and decreased anxiety.

A month into my TV class, I recall looking up on the stage at her assistants and feeling, *I will be there one day!* I was engaged and looking forward to being her student and a student of yoga for life—a commitment that shook me to my core, welled up from an unknown depth of knowing within my fragile body (underweight, inflexible, and depressed). I just knew this yoga was a path I yearned for my whole life.

Recently, as I taught a Zoom class, someone also present that first day, Pat, reminded me of a statement I made to her upon leaving a class one evening. "I am going to be doing this the rest of my life!" And so, it is.

We all walked out, still giggling, and went to the nearby restaurant to eat burgers, fries, and cokes and end the meal with a "much-needed" cigarette. Little did I know that in a few weeks, I would shed these habits naturally and begin a healthier way of living.

Ten-Week Class on Balance, Light and Purpose

A beginners' program consisted of particular yoga asanas and breathing, *pranayama*, for new practitioners to gently unfold their bodies, minds, and hearts. With a careful and methodic way, Lilias offered a practice that respected everyone's challenges. This also included fears and uncertainties studying a foreign exercise and philosophy. This was one of Lilias's gifts. She masterfully created a comfortable environment be it in a school gym in person with rows of yoga students or on TV while she looked into a tiny red light and simplified a vast eastern way of life into a practical, healthy beneficial yoga program for the masses to understand and feel comfortable exploring.

Time magazine dubbed her the "Julia Child of yoga" with a cover story in the early 1970s. PBS markets around the country picked up her show, spotlighting her pointers on alleviating chronic back pain, fatigue, and even how to enhance your golf game. She put Cincinnati, Ohio on the map now for new age studies.

Week after week of consistent practice, one notices changes like a leg lifting a little higher and with less discomfort. The struggle of a sitting forward bend offered a deeper release while my mind became more focused and calmer with proper breathing. One of Lilias's most welcomed moments from us, her students, was her comforting relaxation practices. Her voice was so soothing and when she ended with what felt like a Sanskrit lullaby, chanting the prayer, "Twameva", I slipped through layers into a calming spiritual awakening. It felt like a familiar call to return home. I can still distinctly hear her voice chanting and lulling us into a deep relaxation. I can still feel the presence of a stirring within my heart of hearts for more.

The family and I would leave class exhausted and head to a nearby restaurant to chat it up and smoke. It was the seventies, and no surgeon general warning us not to. However, after only four weeks of yoga practice, when I would light up a cigarette, it would taste terrible and make me cough. It's because yoga asanas correlate their energy alignment with the endocrine system. From the movements and breathing, there is a chemical change and your tongue—with taste—as a chemical reaction would reject the taste of tobacco. After months of deep breathing, pranayama practice, smoking left me naturally after a month of practice. Take note: Four weeks!

Food was another significant change. I ate meat, loved pounding a Swiss steak before cooking it, and began noticing a nausea when smelling meat cooking or raw out of the butcher's package. One evening, while preparing a Swiss steak for our family dinner, I felt an overwhelming nausea and my first thought was, *I'm pregnant again!* Turns out meat was another item for a healthful change, which naturally left me as I continued refining my taste and nervous system through daily yoga practice. This surprised me, and my kids can tell you of my transitioning and theirs into exploring more natural eating of a vegetarian and later, macrobiotic diet. This was never an agenda I entertained or planned.

Into a daily routine now and each evening when the kids were asleep, I came downstairs to my living room and upon a carpet to practice hatha yoga. I had a burning desire to inform my teacher of my deep interest and enthusiasm. I was brutally shy so this would be a major leap of confidence if I could gather the nerve to talk with her after class. I did so with the support of my sister-in-law, Pat. Being accompanied gave me courage. We asked her about learning more regarding meditation. Again, it was her smile and sensing her taking me *in* is how I would express it, to be mentored and set upon a path for the rest of my life. She listened intently to our request of including the study of meditation in the beginner session. And she complied!

An endearing relationship ensued. Lilias recommended reading various books such as *The Gospel of Sri Ramakrishna, Yoga, Youth, and Reincarnation,* and *The Complete Illustrated Book of Yoga,* which I could find at the only new age bookstore, a hole in the wall near the university. Here, I would seek out recommendations, meet other seekers, and try on my first pair of Birkenstock sandals. Also, Lilias gathered some of her friends and students in a spiritual circle to meet at her friend, Bobbie's, house each Wednesday morning to study and discuss. Sometimes, my infant son was included and welcomed in these sessions.

I had no idea where all this movement was headed, but knew within my heart of hearts yoga was truly where I nestled into being who I am. These small spiritual gatherings satisfied a desire to know more at a spiritual level, within its *experiential knowing,* and within pages of *The Bhagavad Gita* and *Upanishads,* I found some solace eventually.

A few other yoga students and I began a meaningful friendship and lovely camaraderie that unlocked other parts of me that were not commiserate with my marriage. What I had been living and what I was gaining in the form of knowledge, alignment and support was like the light of the sun's first strong rays. This didn't translate into action at first, but my awareness channeled awakening.

My friends and I spent hours on our wall phones talking late into the evening about what we were learning and how we were growing. Our children got closer as well. We were all like hungry baby birds, mouths wide open, being fed and chirping wildly about our newfound purpose in life.

At the end of the ten weeks, I had to confront my yearning, or there was no clear next milestone. Could my shy self speak in front of a group and teach? I felt a strength and centeredness I had never experienced before. Depression faded away as a new constant source of balance, lightness and purpose washed over the mundane and anxiety, which had plagued my frail frame. Still. *Teach?* Teaching is modeling. Teaching is leadership. Influential voices helping to heal the world. But I wanted to aid others in transformation like I was experiencing. It's hard to see how far down you've gotten until something you've been craving but didn't have a face reveals itself. I thank God every day for yoga.

Onto the intermediate class, I asked Lilias if I could observe the class on the sidelines for a couple sessions before signing up. This gave my psyche an opportunity to absorb the way Lilias approached the intermediate level, not only from a physical hatha yoga practice but also, what she said during the class. Her explanations were always interesting and immensely helpful to this neophyte. After a couple weeks observing, I signed up for the next session alone. Let's say my family and neighbor had completed their practice. Besides, they were the instruments to get me "there" having signed me up to begin my journey.

My core group were studying, practicing, and exploring a buffet of holistic modalities, leaning on books like Carlos Castaneda's series of *Don Juan* adventures. Somehow these books unfolded another petal of my being with fascination with other realms of reality existing simultaneously. All surged into my inner power and recognizing a connection with all life.

Meet My First Swami

These early days of intermediate yoga study stretched my body into new positions, my mind to new thought patterns, my heart to love and support an even broader community of yoga and holistic practitioners and teachers.

Lilias drove a few of us in her station wagon to Columbus, Ohio where we sat in a small living room and met our first Swami. Not knowing what to expect, we sat crowded, knee to knee, in a space decorated with flowers upon a makeshift altar, statues of deities and offerings of ancient literature. A chair draped in a saffron silk awaited this Swami to appear from another room. He did, to the sounds of all of us chanting interspersed with prayers that felt so natural to me growing up with Latin prayers and songs in Catholic religion. Swamiji Pranananda's bronze skin and striking saffron robe contrasted in a specimen of enchantment and wisdom. I recall one statement from him that I have used in my own teachings: "It doesn't matter if you see colors, a blue or gold or purple light; it doesn't matter if your kundalini rises or falls, this can all be a distraction from your destiny."

He continued, "Yoga is a path to *know* God. To experience the divine nature here and now." This was a head turner for me! Experience God?! After years of Catholic study, I was confused by "we are made in the image and likeness of God" printed within pages of our catechism. Also, the phrase within the "Lord's Prayer", "thy will be done on earth as it is in heaven" spoke to me about the confusion of waiting for another place like heaven when we could feel and be God here and now on earth.

Catholic nuns and priests did their best to answer my young curious mind but always fell short. However, one sister pulled me aside at the end of our school day as we filed in single lines out of the old St. Cecelia school building. It was eighth grade, and my teacher was Sister Mary Alexander. Earlier that day, I had waved my hand in religion class to inquire about yet another memorizing statement from the catechism. She had said she couldn't answer, and I was asked to be seated. Then at the end of the day, she placed her hand on my arm and said, "Diana, this morning in religion class, I want you to know I could not answer your question. But I also want you to know this. Never stop asking questions. Keep inquiring." To this day, I remember and revere Sister Mary Alexander as an important spiritual teacher for me in this lifetime through this one valuable statement from her.

Here was a Swami from India saying God could be experienced here on earth and yoga is a path to experience this. My cells and nervous system were quivering and couldn't wait to hear, to study and experience more. Afterward, I shared with him of my enthusiastic interest to "know" God now. He paused and tapped my heart center a few times, looked into my eyes and said, "Read the book, *How to Know God*. He also said to be in touch with him after I read it.

With Swami's invitation, I felt another layer of guidance and support on this path. This initiated another dimension of yoga study and experience. During our ride home, Lilias's station wagon was filled with lively conversations that lit our imaginations and inquiry all the way down I-71 toward Cincinnati.

The days ahead were laced with excitement. We all gathered at Lilias's house and met her husband, Bob, sons, Michael and Matthew, and their two golden retrievers. Her generous offerings of time and space were invaluable to us and especially to me as I continued upon my journey.

Observing Stars

Nine months into this ecstatic experience, I had dreams of being in front of large groups and teaching. Still suffering mentally and emotionally from shyness and insecurity, I could not even imagine this as a reality before decades of intense effort. However, this pulsation would continue until one day, I finally gathered up courage to mention this to Lilias. Knowing how involved I was with my study, she honored my shyness, and we had many conversations about it.

My mother's illness and death a few years before at the young age of forty-nine seemed to stalk my psyche, involving patterns of aloneness, being orphaned with the loss of my mother's touch, sound of her voice and listening and nurturing. My friend, Carol, who was also studying with another local teacher, encouraged me to write about it as a therapeutic way of processing. I presented the story to *Redbook* magazine, who sent me a genuinely empathetic letter of rejection, encouraging rewrites.

Yoga and its in-depth movement of releasing tensions surfaced and revealed deep-rooted sadness and longings—and my shyness was part of what inhibited the full expression of myself. It was a way of keeping it safely and secretly inside so no one could see it. Note that all the deep pain one has suppressed will begin to surface in a *healthful* way with a wholistic practice of yoga.

As I gathered the courage to tell Lilias of my desire to teach, I was seeing stars on the short walk. No turning back! Again, she listened intently and suggested I teach children first as a way to express verbally and practice seeing into a person practicing. This implied a way of developing a psychic connection and way of "seeing" and teaching. Good idea! I set it up with neighbors and their children that when the school bus pulled up with wild energy of kids who sat in desks pretty much all day, I would offer a yoga class to exercise and calm them. Only one neighbor refused, as her church felt I needed saving because of practicing yoga. (Ironic, since my life couldn't be more SAVED!) Everyone else welcomed the idea and the class began.

My kids, Angie, Jamie, and Brad, along with their neighborhood friends, hopped off the school bus and headed to our family room. We practiced a few yoga stretches emulating animals and having fun in "cobra sticking out snake tongues", "growling in a lion pose", "shaky tree balances" and at end of the twenty-minute session, a deep relaxation. To my astonishment, they were still in Sarvasana as I guided them with visuals of floating upon clouds with soft smiles upon their face, soft eyes, and hearts. It was a success and word got around, so I was invited to teach a few minutes at end of the school day at the elementary school.

Lilias was becoming increasingly popular and traveled, teaching throughout the country and appearing on national TV shows. Her expertise in relating an ancient practice from India to modern-day America was a gift for many. Worldwide, people were taking notice of the PBS TV star's unique offerings for feeling better at home, work and while on the go. Practical yoga was beneficial for everyone. Because of her continued classes in Cincinnati, she would need subs from time to time. Still working through some layers of insecurity, I would not qualify to teach a crowded gym of adults and who all came to learn from a famous TV personality. Now, that would be so intimidating.

But it happened.

She asked if I would sub one day. Several of us had been

assisting and suggesting ways of entering poses with Lilias's eye of approval. We never pushed. As I assisted students, I learned to articulate through whispering cues without even touching. I was amazed at the results. I was now an official assistant like the two women on stage who I noticed that first night.

Now I was to teach and lead my first official adult class and did so, nervously entering the room that evening, yet knowing, *I've got this*. Two of my yoga buddies sat beside me assisting and with their support and generosity as I taught my first adult yoga session. I was hoping the students were not too disappointed in not being with Lilias. I assured them I understood if they were, and I would do my best in sharing what she had taught me.

Within the first few moments of speaking, I was well into my "seeing" and being with each individual and entire class. The yoga asanas, the breathing, pranayama and the final relaxation and meditation I guided with ease and a deep familiarity. I even recited the lovely "Twameva" chant. Not a moment of timidity appeared. I was relieved at the end to receive gracious feedback and hugs acknowledging me as a yoga teacher. I received comments regarding how soothing my voice was, which had been my ultimate test. I have never looked back.

REACH AND RECEIVE: REMEMBER WHAT LIGHTS YOU UP

Reflect on the beginning of a life experience that inspires you to this day. If you are a yoga teacher, recall your first day entering a class, being mentored, being inspired. Whatever your calling, recalling your first steps upon your path is a memory that lights up your journey. Let it continue to be remembered as your initiation in this lifetime of finding your true path. Let's honor and respect all our unique journeys. After all, as Ram Dass says, "We are all just walking each other home."

Chapter 2

Spirit Calls and Awakens a New Depth

"Only those who will risk going too far can possibly find out how far one can go."

—T.S. Elliott

A DEEPER CALLING AWAKENED me each morning hungry to know more, to experience more and to become a yogi, as those who I read and studied. I recall reading books of saints and popes as a young Catholic girl looking for inspiration. Now, as an adult, I read of saints of another culture and philosophy. I so wanted to find a specific practice to experience God/the Divine Mystery here and now on earth. A yogi was one who dedicated their life to know experientially throughout their whole being a divine purpose and connection.

I reflect on the initiatory process of becoming a yogi. A new step in this process of deepening, expanding, and experiencing was through weekend yoga retreats.

My first retreat took place in Columbus, Ohio with Swami Pranananda, who became my spiritual teacher and guide. It was my first experience devoting an entire weekend to yoga practice. Sleep the night before turned into the stars on my ceiling twinkling with possibility. Who needed sleep after being in another kind of rest from fully living? I was jumping out of my skin anticipating the morning hours. A whirlwind of change accelerated within my body. My circuitry charged with a current of curiosity, which I also recall feeling as a young child in the Catholic church as we attended mandatory mass almost daily.

In those early days at St. Cecelia, we all attended morning mass as a class. I wanted to prove to God I really wanted to know and be with Him, so I would walk a mile in the dark hours to a 6:30 a.m. mass attended by a few elderly women and men of the parish and me. It felt more sincere and sacred in some way. The dimly lit church and deep quietude nourished me in some way too.

Sitting in silence in front near Swami's feet, we listened to his talks on the studies of yoga and ways to apply teachings within our everyday lives. I was impressed by the psychology of yoga, a vast system so ancient yet so applicable to modern-day psychology and physiology studies. I recall vibrant conversations with Jan, a psychologist and yoga student friend, about how yoga felt so comprehensive in its layers of understanding the human condition. Pure, accessible healing energy.

The darshan talks with Swamiji were balanced with an intense hatha yoga session morning and afternoon with Sita Frenkel from the New York seminary/ashram. Sita was a tough taskmaster, and we would feel any and all tension wrung out of our bodies. We would be so sore the next day and the thought of practicing in a class again was sometimes dreadful. But we were better for it.

On the last day, Sunday, I asked Swamiji, a resident monk in a New York ashram, if he would consider coming to Cincinnati. He agreed! I was so delighted to have this opportunity for our community and not a clue as to how to put this whole event together. But I knew it was to be and I was to create this. Lilias guided my enthusiastic intentions into a practical plan of execution, and others got involved as well. We did it! I am not sure of the timing between attending my first retreat to creating a retreat, but the journey was one I dove into with all my heart. I believe it was from a space of spring to fall the same year, spanning preparation, logistics and the fervor of the community to pull this off. It had been an amazing weekend with many from out of town in the Midwest attending, and the rooms all filled with eager, helpful participants sharing the path.

One beautiful memory is walking out in afternoon to the lush green pine grove at Grailville, the retreat center, for Satsang with Swamiji. As I slowly and reverently entered the shaded area, pine needles cushioned our mats, and the scent of the fresh pine opened the senses to internalize teachings more readily in a more somatic absorption. The contrast of Swami's saffron-colored, layered robes with the vibrant green pine tree, is still a sensual memory of this wonderful spiritual moment. I can walk into the pine grove and remember it today. Someone asked him why the "orange-colored" robes. He responded, "The saffron color represents the fire of renunciation and the light of wisdom."

We practiced hatha yoga a couple times a day taught by Sita. She was such a sweet yet intimidating presence. We all wanted to be as far away from the front of room because she would always use a student near her to demonstrate. Holding a cobra pose while Sita thoroughly instructed with precise pointers was so challenging.

One's body would literally tremble. I was one of those students and learned so much from her. I recall holding a pose in front of our retreatants while she detailed the alignment, the areas supporting for strength, the benefits. This seemed like hours as I steadfastly attempted to remain within the boundaries of the yoga asana.

After the release, she looked at me with a smile and asked, "So, did you see God?" Everyone laughed. Because of the intensity, I sure thought I was on my way off the earth and into His arms!

The silent meditation sessions early morning and late evening were placed at maximum hours to embrace the divine nature of our retreat days. Meals were important nutrition for our bodies and minds, as well as the community participation in preparation and cleanup. We all did so with such joy and devotion rather than a dreaded discipline. We were enlisted alphabetically, which ensured you would be with people you were meeting from around the country for the first time and sharing your story and enthusiasm for yoga. Grailville was notorious for an excellent quality of food and oh, the homemade bread aroma and taste. The yum of yoga retreating in those days!

Grailville retreat center in Loveland, Ohio, was the mainstay for this retreat and many more to follow throughout the decades. It was the place to experience a solo silent retreat, a group yoga retreat, a place to visit on one's own to walk the beautiful grounds, purchase spiritual books, gifts, and incense in their on-point gift shop. Best of all, it was only twenty minutes from my home. I brought in Christian mystic healer Rev. Carol Parrish, who Lilias had introduced me to, and other yogis from around the world like Bernard Rishi from France and Karin Stephan from Boston to lead retreats.

With a couple of these locally sponsored retreats within the second year of my yoga practice, Lilias encouraged me to go to study during weekends and a week-long training at the yoga seminary in Harriman, New York. Somehow with young children at home, I managed to cover all my bases, including expenses, and head out to the Yoga Seminary of New York for deep dives into yoga. There, I befriended many from across the country who were as eager and hungry for more. This comprehensive study included rigorous hatha yoga twice daily with Sita, yoga philosophy with Hans, Sita's husband and yoga philosophy teacher, and spiritual discourse with Swami Pranananda.

When I think back on this time at this ashram nestled in the Catskill Mountains, totally immersed in yoga teachings, how blessed I am today for this rich, fulfilling experience. And I have Lilias to be grateful for nudging me upon a path she knew was authentic and valuable to my maturing as a *teacher*.

Initiation

My now many layered yoga experiences inspired a desire to be initiated into yoga. Initiation was the receiving of a blessing, *Shaktipat*, from one's teacher/mentor. It was the infusion of spiritual current of grace. In so many of these teachings I was reading and listening to in person, this ceremony sparked my longing in another way. Growing up Catholic I was very inspired and knowledgeable about the initiations through the holy sacraments. The holy waters at baptism, the holy eucharist at first communion, the oils and receiving a name at confirmation were very special moments in my spiritual journey.

This was no different. It wasn't leaving something else to take on another cloak of consciousness but felt purposeful to receive for my spiritual journey to continue. I approached Lilias regarding this, and we both concluded it would be appropriate time to ask Swamiji Pranananda for such an experience. I had been with him now for a couple of years in person and corresponding. Although, I must say still something just didn't feel it was the right person. However, I did approach him, and he listened with deep, respectful attention and proceeded to tap my heart while pronouncing prayers. He placed his gentle palm upon my head and blessed the current of reaching and receiving I was requesting. I was honored and walked away feeling fulfilled in some way.

I later came to the realization and went to Lilias with my new request. She listened as I spoke of my experience with Swamiji, was happy it happened, but I told her there was more. I realized though this was meaningful in some way, it was she, Lilias, who I felt my journey reached for this initiation sacrament to receive. We both prayed upon this, and it happened!

I showed up at her lovely home with a bouquet of yellow mums, eager to receive and share this sacred energetic experience with her. It was, indeed, a sacred moment. I received my mantra and so much more!

Lilias gifted me her prayer shawl to wear when I meditate, which I have still in my room. She also surprised me with a very special gift, a guitar! Lilias knew how much I enjoyed leading chanting in classes and retreats and often saying I wish I knew how to play guitar. This moment, my intuition to complete the initiation process with her and with Swamiji, continues to deepen and inspire my journey.

REACH AND RECEIVE:
SILENT RETREATS

Pause and create moments of healing silence feeling the breath at the tip of your nose flow gently in/out. Cluttered, rambling thoughts will eventually disappear, and your mind will be relaxed and clear. Your focus of attention will increase without stress gradually as days go by. Choose a day to let go of distractions (even music playing). It gives your nervous system a breather. It is so soothing for your health and wellbeing. Silent retreats can be so nourishing and a way to reconnect with your Sacred Source! Give yourself this opportunity. It could be an adventure with a tent-camping experience in the forest where you feel into the quiet sustenance of nature. Simply take a walk where the sounds of a city are not heard, and permit the natural sounds of birds, breezes, tree leaves rustling, a babbling brook or waterfall soothe your body-mind-heart.

Chapter 3

Silence: The Ultimate Teacher

"When you arise in the morning, think of what a precious privilege it is to be alive-to breathe, to think, to enjoy, to love."

—Marcus Aurelius

A S IT HAPPENED, Swamiji Chidananda, head of the Ramakrishna order of monks from Rishikesh was going to be visiting the seminary in New York. With lots of preparation on my homefront, my husband dropped me off at Lilias's home and Bob, her husband, drove us to the airport. I still recall Bob's conversations about Swamiji Chidananda, who he had met many times before. He spoke of his deep respect for this Swami and how he was the real deal. I realized in some way his words were preparing me for my first encounter with a holy man.

I flew with Lilias to spend the weekend at this seminary and meet the head of the Ramakrishna order of monks. Sitting near me now as I write this, is a small booklet created from a talk he gave one eve during this very retreat. It was on silence. I recall sitting beside Lilias in a candle-lit room, the fragrance of fresh flowers upon the altar in the design of the sacred sound of *Om*, and the soft chanting of all who attended this weekend. We sat in silence for a while, and he began to softly speak on the value of silence and realizing our divine nature. We all had tears streaming down our cheeks while he gently spoke, and the sound of his words seemed to touch and affect each and every one of us within our hearts. I remember feeling, *this is a man who experiences the Divine as saints have. He speaks from that vibration. This must be what Shaktipat is!*

I felt I was in the presence of someone, something much greater and touched my heart with grace. I felt I was in the presence of a living saint! I could write chapters of this meeting alone as it was a sacred magnificent moment in my ever-evolving spiritual life. Here is an excerpt of Swamiji's talk, darshan with a saint, I say!

"Beloved and blessed children of light! The real, ultimate teaching is silence. The real teaching is simply silence. It is not to utter words. Words and speech constitute a human phenomenon. Human nature and all its movements are finite and limited. …All speech implies duality."

Explaining the value and limitations of words in knowing God, Supreme Consciousness, and how ancient scriptures, the written word, is still confined to time, space, name, and form, he said words may direct us with ingredients for a mystical experience but cannot in and of themselves be the ultimate immersive divine consciousness.

Swamiji spoke with a current that electrified the room with a divine light Source and held our untamed, wild minds and bodies with a stillness and peaceful calm I can feel this day as I write. We were touching new realms of silence in our stillness. I recall another comment from this dear, saintly teacher. One evening, when he arrived for evening *satsang* (truth in the gathering of spiritual friends), after a few minutes of quiet reflection, he opened his soft eyes, looked around as if to take us all into his sacred heart, and seeing most of us clad in our newly purchased prayer shawls, mala beads in hands, he commented we needn't take on another way to pray with all its accessories. We need not leave our religion to enter yoga spiritual teachings. Yoga is like the spectacle {glasses} we use to see Truth within any religion or spiritual pathway.

As this weekend continued to deepen in teaching experiences, I began valuing even more the powerful rituals, sacraments of Catholicism. It was a swami from India who ignited this appreciation and respect within me. I am forever grateful! I felt I was touched by grace experientially for the first time.

For a couple years, I and my yoga teacher friend, Jill, would attend and study in-depth yoga teachings at Yoga Seminary of New York and return to share with fellow teachers and students. Also, Sita and Swamiji Pranananda would travel to Cincinnati and Columbus, Ohio as they now had quite an enthusiastic Midwest following and interest. I am so deeply fond of these days, these special teachers and teachings, the fellow yogi students I met and loved along the way. It provided me with a secure foundation and pathway of knowledge from which I can steadily and sturdily walk upon and retrieve the "Light of Wisdom" from one saintly man in a saffron robe.

These years of enthusiastic study created a foundation not only of in-depth knowledge of yoga and its branches of philosophical wisdom but brought forth a courage and self-esteem within my frail and battered ego. Shyness to speak in public settings to groups slowly subsided and peeled away from my frame. I became confident and passionate more and more while teaching in groups both small and large.

One special moment in time, Lilias offered two different experiences to me. The first would be giving a presentation at a local Catholic institution. St. Joseph Infant Home requested Lilias give an experiential talk to staff. She was unable due to timing so offered this yoga "gig" to me. *Whoa!* This would be my first formal talk in front of a group besides our yoga classes. I was nervous yet excited! It was for the women's guild of the infant home.

I entered the room ready with a basic idea of how to have the staff and women practice yoga and reap some benefits. To my surprise, I walked into the event and there was a room filled with nuns with full dress layers including habits and veils atop their heads! What could I possibly do here? This would be my first exercise in improvising and creating a new yoga experience. I spoke a little of benefits of a simple yoga practice with breathing and spinal movements and relaxation. While they were sitting in metal folding chairs, I grabbed one also and began moving with hatha yoga in a chair, had them reaching underneath the veils and massaging their scalps, tapping their arms, chest, and legs with Do-In massage. Yoga teachers had just experienced a workshop with Bernard Rishi from France and Karin Stephan, an Iyengar teacher from Boston who accompanied him and shared this energizing technique, and a few *pranayama*, breaths they could practice to relieve stress and create calm. I led the group through a deep relaxation/meditation into the cave of their heart. And here, "chair yoga" began in the mid-1970s! Creative improvisation in certain circumstances is my forte. I enjoy the challenge to this day.

When all was said and done, the response was overwhelmingly appreciative and grateful. Individuals coming up and thanking and sharing their experiences was so heartwarming. The head of the guild approached me, thanking me and presenting a votive candle in a beautiful glass holder—my first payment for teaching, which I still have today! I treasure the little candle as a reminder of a significant moment on the path of my vocation. Teaching at a Catholic facility with a group of sisters/nuns was a familiar setting from my childhood and it seemed I had come full circle, a sacred circle in some way. My heart was full, and I could not wait to share the experience with Lilias.

Another exciting gift was traveling with Lilias to Sarasota, Florida for a yoga retreat she was to teach sponsored by Rev. Carol Parrish, a Christian mystic, healer, psychic who I was introduced to by Lilias earlier in the year. Lilias and Carol invited me to attend and assist her during this event. Well, with her popularity now on a national level with her successful TV program, "Lilias, Yoga and You", the retreat was overflowing with participants! The hotel auditorium was filled with eager participants who wanted to meet and study with Lilias. Because of the size of the crowd, it was decided to have all yoga teachers who had traveled from around the state in another room and the yoga students stay in this room. It was then decided to split up the teaching; I in one room and Lilias in the other! Now mind you, this was quite exciting yet intimidating. These enthusiastic students and teachers wanted to be with Lilias. So, it was decided, I would go to the room with teachers and instruct while she would remain in the large hall with students. We then would switch off in afternoon session.

My heart could probably be noticed beating rapidly through my yellow leotard with anxiety over entering a room full of teachers who I felt were disappointed Lilias was not there. I took a deep breath, walked into the room of yoga teachers from around the south and began teaching. I recall asking them what, if anything, did they desire to learn that day. I listened intently and began offering in a most humble way what I felt they may be interested in. I also invited them, as teachers, to freely inquire with questions. This dissolved any insecurity on my part and seemed to soften the initial disappointment of not having Lilias with them.

I started out telling them I know they wanted traveled to be with Lilias and assured them they would be in the afternoon. I shared my background and then began to instruct how to approach a beginning student and class. I presented poses and contraindication possibilities and found myself diving in with passion and drawing up knowledge from within my experience now of a couple of years. The two hours or so flew by. At the end, I guided a deep relaxation. I was tearfully grateful at their kind and generous responses afterward and what the instruction meant to them. *Whew!* Yet another new experience where I was thrown into the waters and swam to shore!

As we all went to a lunch break, I walked up to a smiling Lilias and was embraced in a loving, caring moment of relief as I shared my experience and survival.

In the afternoon, we switched off, and I now sat in front of room filled with yoga students. I talked briefly and separated those with more experience. I continued leading them through a beginner's series of poses and breath work, while including some intermediate variations for the more experienced students. It also went very well and at the end, I guided them through a calming relaxation. I received glowing comments at the end, which gave me more confidence for my future endeavors.

I was overflowing with gratitude as I sat at the end of the day workshop beside Lilias and Carol on stage and felt the familiar soothing nurturing response in my body while Lilias chanted the Sanskrit prayer, "Twameva", the lullaby-like song I first heard years ago in a school gym during my first yoga class. I have come full circle once again and felt initiated on a path of my vocation, my purpose for being here this lifetime.

That evening, we celebrated at a beautiful outdoor feast. Some of the yoga teachers who were students of Carol's teachings of Christian mysteries were there, along with Swami Muktananda's students. This swami would also be an influence in my life and teaching though I did not know this at that moment. Carol presented me with a book as a birthday gift, *The Masters and the Path*, by Charles Webster Leadbeater. I cherished this moment for so many reasons. This gift opened my psyche to experience even more in-depth teachings of the sacred. I was being introduced to esoteric teachings, which unfolded the mystic in me. Mystics, too, had been fascinating to me as a young Catholic girl.

This trip to Florida with Lilias would have a dramatic impact on my life going forward in so many ways. Thank you, dear Lilias and Carol, for your trust and confidence in me and most especially for the deep, nurturing of this fledgling while she grew her wings to fly!

Chapter 4

Healers of The Grail

"We have a tendency to think in terms of doing and not in terms of being. We think that when we are not doing anything, we are wasting our time. But that is not true. Our time is, first of all, for us to be. To be what? To be alive, to be peaceful, to be joyful, to be loving. And that is what the world needs most."

—THICH NHAT HANH

GRAILVILLE WAS HOME to The Grail, an international women's movement and a well-known spiritual oasis just outside of Cincinnati. The many acres of land tended to by the wide range of women from far around the world included lush organic gardens, dairy cow pastures, and housing buildings with such unique architectural structures, including the award-winning Oratory, a beautiful, sacred space that fills my heart each time I enter. I can still hear the hundreds of voices that chanted and sang, the many yogis, including myself, being taught by various. The sweat and tears of sadness, emotional releases, and great joy, which expressed throughout these walls, still reverberate from

41

the wooden beams. The natural sunlight rays piercing through the sun window on roof illuminates the altar upon which many universal rituals, prayers and meditations were expressed throughout the decades. This revered space feels like a familiar friend to me when I walk into the opulent room. I am flooded with wondrous spiritual yoga memories.I vividly recall the retreat I sponsored with Christian mystic and teacher Rev. Carol Parrish. By the time I sponsored Carol, I had been under her tutelage and was so impressed with her knowledge of esoteric teachings, which included yoga. She would return a few times to Cincinnati to lead spiritual retreats and had quite a following of interested aspirants in yoga and an array of other teachings and studies. I would return to Sarasota and study many levels of development within the chakras, such as the psychic development using her teacher's mystical teaching tool of the Shustah cards. I have many profound experiences with this and other tools to use to unfold my layers of knowing and experiencing. One I share always is "tapping" your pituitary gland lightly to stimulate your psychic ability to "see".

When in Loveland, Ohio at Grailville during a particular retreat, Carol led us through esoteric teachings of the chakras from both yoga and other traditions. It was so intriguing how she wove various threads of worldly teachings together for a more complete understanding and honor of all esoteric paths as one. Also, during this particular retreat, in her Southern accent, she gently guided us through a past-life regression exercise. I recall lying there upon my yoga mat in the Oratory building and having a jumbled list of things I needed to do as director of the retreat rambling on in my mind. I felt I would not be able to follow her guidance but was glad the filled room of participants lying upon their mats with blanketed comfort would experience this provocative meditative regression exercise.

Then *poof*! I recall her saying look at your feet (this is with eyes closed in meditation} and mine were bare, dark-skinned, and dusty. The sensation of the soft dirt on my soles was so palpable and she continued to guide us to eventually see our whole self and environment. There I was an Indian squaw, young, centered and confident in who I was. This exercise continued and I can assure you it was a moment that awakened my ability to shapeshift, something I would soon discover through Castaneda writings.

Another significant moment during this retreat at Grailville with Carol was an introduction for many of us to an annual Buddhist sacred event/holy day, Wesak Festival. Since this retreat fell on the full moon in Taurus in May, Carol asked me if I thought it was appropriate to share this event through ritual. I fully honored her ability to introduce it in a way that was welcoming to all and so, she gave me a list of items and instructions of how to set up the altar for this event. A beautiful punch bowl filled with water, candles, incense, prayer cloths and explicit placement for each item.

We all entered the candlelit room in the evening and with the full moon light rays through the solar panels upon the altar and reflecting in the water, well, it was one of the most aesthetically gorgeous and powerful esoteric moments I can recall. Carol proceeded to share this event as a lovely story of the Buddha and his return celebrated during this full moon for centuries. It was a moment where and when the veil is lifted, and you experience the great heart and mind of the Buddha. Now mind you, Carol is a Christian mystic who is sharing this and weaves into the story how the Christ and Buddha are known as brothers in esoteric teachings. The moment the storyline ended and the sacred silence began was impressive and inspiring to all!

The veil lifts and you are in a cellular communication with a vibration so astounding, so light filled you are impressed for the rest of your life! "Thy will be done on earth as it is in heaven," says Christ.

My dear friend who reads this now, you who are taking yoga classes or in one of the many yoga teacher trainings, I urge you to jump out of only attending/teaching one-hour classes at gyms or studios, go attend retreats. Dive into sacred silence where your greatest teacher awaits you! Seek those who *know* esoteric wisdom, not just spouting from books but from *living experience*. The sacred *shaktipat* is an energy exchange which will enlighten and awaken your own true self! Just as holy sacraments I received in Catholicism, so have I received from the wisdom and energy exchange of great teachers.

Within your sacred heart of hearts, you will rest in the wisdom and love which shall sustain you for all your life. This truly is where *"thy will be done on earth as it is in heaven"* resides.

REACH AND RECEIVE: FEEL THE EARTH IN YOUR PRACTICE

Explore beyond the realm of confined rooms and allow the earth's beauty and spacious landscapes to inspire a deep unfolding of yourself. Your yoga and somatic movement practice will flourish and be nourished in ways that await your arrival. Just breathe and jump into the unknown!

Chapter 5

Seven Yogis with a Vision: Birth of CYTA

"Go out into the world today and love the people you meet. Let your presence light new light in the hearts of people."

—MOTHER TERESA

THERE WAS A new age bookstore located near the University of Cincinnati, New World bookstore, run by Ed Kluska, a local astrologer and friend to all in the new age community. In the 1970s, Cincinnati, Ohio was a bustling hub for well-grounded new age ideas, philosophies, and practices. Most all involved would eventually meet up or be introduced to each other through Ed, who also owned the New World food shop, which included a small dining area of all vegetarian items. This was our source also for knowledge of nutrients and his manager, Sherry T. was very knowledgeable and adept at providing abundant information and suggestions, all which were so helpful for me. She and I would become good friends and even traveled together for a health convention in Santa Monica.

45

Can you imagine there were only a handful of books regarding yoga? No Google searches! A few books I still have included *The Complete Illustrated Book of Yoga*, by Swami Vishnudevananda, whose ashram was nearby the Yoga Seminary of New York located in the Catskills Mountains. Sita, the teacher who I mentioned earlier, also wrote a hatha yoga text, which was available for her students and teachers. Lilias, of course, also through her PBS series on yoga, published a companion book, *Lilias, Yoga and You*. These three texts were my main resource at the time and provided excellent reference for hatha yoga studies. While on the subject of books, I will note at the ashram/seminary in New York, I also gathered books from India written on science of yoga by Sivananda and other yoga scholars and medical doctors. These books were so instructive on science of pranayama breathing, and many aspects of yoga philosophical studies including the sutras and the *Bhagavad Gita*. I have still in my unique and vast library of yoga and new age teachings, educational materials including these very texts from India.

As I mentioned, at the beginning there were many attending Lilias's yoga classes and with her PBS TV series there were teachers popping up here and there across the city and of course, around the country. Many of us would attend a variety of classes, experiencing different styles and methods and began seeing each other for visits at lunch and other social gatherings. It sparked with a conversation and then a meeting at a friend of Lilias and yoga teacher Sheila Bading's house. A handful of new teachers including myself who were following different teachers around the Ohio, Indiana, Kentucky region met. We all had a desire to enjoin in some way or fashion, for community and a way to pull our resources to conduct ongoing educational opportunities and teacher trainings.

This moment in the 1970s, Cincinnati Yoga Teachers Association (CYTA) was birthed and evolved into a vibrant community of teachers and yoga enthusiasts from the tri-state area, Ohio, Kentucky, and Indiana. We boasted a lawyer, accountant, insurance agent, and artist (designing our logo) all teaching yoga aiding and contributing their professional career expertise in the business aspect of forming a non-profit association. My manual typewriter was the source of typing out our bylaws, according to *Robert's Rules for Organization*, as well as newsletters to all members and the community-wide new age enthusiasts. We became the hub for all information regarding events in the area. This was a very exciting time. During this moment of organizing, we selected ourselves to be in various board member positions to enable a better professional face of our community. We worked countless hours, coalescing over phone time each day, then met each week in person with more developing ideas and business details. And this was not an easy process by any means. It was full-on dedication to the creative idea, its unfolding into the process of becoming and finally, manifestation.

We were ready to hold our first meeting and invited so many contacts throughout the Midwest to attend. We held the first election of board members with nominations from various members giving reasons why their "candidate" would be so honored to hold a position. My dear friend, Jan Kolish, nominated me to my surprise, gave a beautiful talk, it was seconded, and I was chosen through voting by my peers to be the first duly elected president of CYTA!

I was tearfully appreciative and dove in 100% with a wonderful expert-filled board of directors to ride this wave into the new age! We surged with creating a plethora of yoga workshops and even created a soon-to-be popular Day of Yoga presentation. This Day of Yoga included four sessions lasting a little over hour with a lunch break. It included presenting teachers from a variety of venues in yoga and other modalities of holistic health. Each session offered a few options you could choose from, would check off and send in with your check. These were sold-out events!

This venue began to include massage therapists, healers of various modalities, and bookstore vendors such as Victor Paruta of Victory Light bookstore in Covington, Kentucky. Meditation, chanting, Iyengar yoga, beginner yoga, intermediate yoga, philosophy, tai chi, and so many other modalities filled Day of Yoga. It was a great way to advertise your own unique teaching and it was *the* event of the year in Cincinnati and tri-state area for the entire new age community. We would rent out high schools, the YMCA, and other venues for the event. CYTA quickly dominated the map as a valuable resource for education and community. I couldn't be prouder of what a handful of yogis in a living room who had a vision manifested as a great community service for education, social, community—our three pillars which are present today!

Also, CYTA helped other organizations nationally and internationally organize as we had the proven working formula for a non-profit yoga business and vibrant community. We brought in renowned international teachers of Iyengar yoga, the Himalayan Institute, medical doctors who were yogis, spiritual teachers, and local doctors who gave presentations, such as the famous Dr. Robert Fulford, who was my physician and that of a few other yoga teachers. His cranial sacral work, which aided so many, consisted of the technique of sensating and supporting the subtle movement of cranial sutures and the respiratory movement, and simply the important flexing of your feet to stimulate organs and glands.

Another time we sponsored him together with Dr. Frédérick Leboyer, *Birth without Violence* author and instructor from France. After a lecture at Xavier University, the two visited a small yoga studio owned by yoga teacher Winnie Denny and proceeded to guide us through the cranial sacral work and its importance to vibrant health! We also learned how important the birthing environment is for both the mother and baby. His book added visuals to the process of water birthing. Dr. Fulford contributed with his cranial/sacral therapy important information and data referring to the trauma of sutures being utilized and how delicate one must be with touch and holding and shaping of the baby's head. We learned how so many of the baby's movements effect the brain's development and are like yoga moves. How fortunate for our community to have Dr. Fulford and so many gifted healers and teachers in our presence! Acclaimed holistic physician, Dr. Andrew Weil, was fortunate enough to bring Dr. Fulford to Arizona where he was respected as a known healer. I am so blessed to have been taught cranial sacral therapy hands-on by this remarkable physician and healer. More importantly, I was privileged to be a patient receiving his healing knowledge and touch! I can still feel his gentle hands releasing deep tensions and receiving the gifts this inspiring doctor and teacher shared selflessly.

The list of teachers and trainings CYTA brought to the area were funded through our annual dues of just $35 and from the revenue we received from the many sold-out events throughout the years. We also held an annual dinner sometimes with an expert's presentation such as Dr. Tom Bender, an orthopedic surgeon with his slides of spine and joints and contraindications. Dr. Jack Armstrong, DC, was a favorite presenter of nutrition and anatomical guidance as well. We all were immersed in continued study and dedicated to being the knowledgeable teachers guiding others on their path of wellness. Dr. Swami Amritananda, affiliated with Integral Yoga, oversaw a weekend of intense anatomy, physiology and philosophy studies pertaining to yoga. We were presented with an endocrinology curriculum of study pertaining to the energy centers known in yoga as chakras. The science studies from the Himalayan Institute presented to us from Swami Rama, and Dr. Robert Benson, of the *Relaxation Response* book were also included in our studies with in-person educational events.

The decorated list goes on. Donna Farhi, a contemporary teacher to many throughout the world, became a friend, and I am glad to see her continue to espouse an intelligent and respectful approach to yoga. Jean Couch is another dear friend in yoga who came to instruct Iyengar-style yoga with its precise alignment and delightfully without the rigidity but rather, with humor and lightness! Many of us who were studying Iyengar style back in the day were subject to few teachers who seemed ruthless. Such a blessing to have had Jean Couch and others showing the more feminine way of approaching alignment. Oh, yes, there is such a "way". Jean's brilliance and enthusiasm continue to inspire my teaching and study.

In Cincinnati, back many decades ago, we paved a very wide pathway for the new age community to explore and continue with depth and enthusiasm and most of all, respect and friendship. My gratitude to all the teachers back in the day, many who have left this earth, some my very dear friends who I continue to miss and love! Jan Kolish and Jill Robb McConnell were two close friends and instrumental in the dissemination of yoga teaching in the region. To this day, I miss them tremendously. I look forward to playing with Jan and Jill in another place, another time, another realm of time and space.

As of this writing, this week is a memorial to Roger Null, one of our seven seekers for community in that living room in the early 70s. Roger, the truck driver who became a yoga teacher, was a popular instructor with his practical and passionate discourses on yoga. His contribution to the dissemination of yoga is tremendous. A dear friend I will miss and draw upon for continued inspiration. My three yogi angels, Jan, Jill, and Roger, I salute you!

There are other teachers as well who offered selflessly for the cause of disseminating yoga as a vibrant healing practice and gave valued time and effort for the community created with CYTA. Mary Louise Kemper and Jenny Luken were dear friends and companions along the way.

REACH AND RECEIVE: LEGACY

Are you a part of a yoga practice or healing community? Share your knowledge and resources. Seek out those who may aid and draw visibility to your region. You never know who may need a group or ready service today! Remember the power of your contribution and that of a handful of people wanting to change the world from their living rooms!

Chapter 6

Gurus Galore

"The purpose of yoga is to stop the misery before it comes."

—Patanjali

THE BEATLES POPULARIZED the experience of being in the presence of a guru while practicing transcendental meditation with Maharishi Mahesh. It seemed so many men in various communities were popularizing this experience and creating followers, filling a spiritual void or perhaps by exploiting the followers' naivete. I say this with honoring the selfless, caring teachers who are dedicated in a vocation to share what they know and be enthused for their students to create their own path.

Yoga was becoming more popular and there were teachers who were looking for followers. Seemed to be an abundance of both. I was introduced to Swami Muktananda in the late 1970s and was impressed with the dynamic flow of energy I experienced while in meditation using the mantra imparted by him to the seekers. It just so happened to be the same mantra given to me during Initiation a few years earlier.

When I arrived home, I discovered a group of his students in Cincinnati and would attend their Sunday eve chanting sessions along with other hatha yoga teachers and many others who gathered for this communal meditation experience. I love chanting since a child, so this all was a familiar and lovely experience for me. I met wonderful new friends there too. Always open to widen the community.

Rajneesh was another yogi guru who had published writings, which I found to be profoundly moving me into deeper experiences of meditation. His prose deepened my understanding of mysteries and impressed my psyche into a new way of expressing using specific verbiage within the context of my teaching. I was never in his presence but did find his writings to be inspiring. His teachings included living fully and knowing you already are a god-being on earth. His take on renunciation was different as he felt all experiences were beautiful and to be enjoyed. This was controversial with many teachings as renunciation and celibacy was a needed power for some to attain your God experience.

When I was in a presence of a guru type, always I would feel into the experiences with wide open curiosity and safeguarding when it just felt like a line of guru BS! And I can say, this happened with a few to be sure. I need not to speak of their names or circumstances for it has dissolved into the ethers for me, but I can say I personally know sincere seekers who were bamboozled into giving up homes and livelihoods with families to follow them. Here, I take a deep breath as I recall the manipulation. And almost always with these characters, their so-called teachings that included trashing other modalities and teachers/teachings. This is always a "red flag"! Tantric yoga is probably the most misunderstood and misused teachings for manipulative circumstances.

Sexual exploitations under the guise of teaching how to handle sexual energy flow is nothing new either. And it certainly isn't privy just to yoga dudes. We are all aware of various sexual dishonor in religions, schools and with trusted officials in power.

Hatha yoga also has been exploited by well-known male teachers who use their female students to act out through inappropriate touching in the guise of correcting a pose. There are more avenues of righting this horrible wrong occurring especially with the MeToo movement! Expelled teachers from ashrams and yoga studio closings have increased simply due to this atrocious misuse and abuse of yoga teaching. Standards are continually being written into bylaws throughout the world regarding safety of students in many layers of body-mind-heart study. This is why even in the 1970s, our Cincinnati Yoga Association was valuable in promoting and honoring decency and respect and calling on the carpet when any abuse was found. It was a well-respected entity where one could seek out help in many ways.

This is not just relegated to yoga obviously; many religions seek to have people follow a preacher and tithe your income whilst they live in luxurious mansions or religious complexes. Today, this continues and melds into other areas of life such as politics. Narcissistic characters looking to manipulate and be adored is nothing new or just old. "If you see something, say something" applies with relevancy to yoga teachers too! Reach out to well-known and well-respected teachers and seek their guidance and support. We are here for you!

In this new millennium, do you feel into the experience of real authentic yoga teachers with a lineage of energetic wisdom and light? Are the teacher training programs that are being produced en masse nowadays for yoga careers securing profitable income for studios and persons the new falsehood fakirs? Meaning, their few weekend lessons secure a certification and then those who receive this also offering teacher trainings for profit at the expense of in-depth experience and knowledge from a lineage of many years, decades, and practice, as well as sharing with others. In truth, we must take a look at this honestly and lay down our yoga mats, blocks, clothing attire and feel into what is real and unreal about this in regards to yoga. Everyone must examine their own participation in whatever way to continue the promotion of yoga under the guise of flashy marketing and materials/products.

Most of the guru types are male with the exception of very few women. Most popular and known today is Mata, also known as Amma. Her devotees are aligned in bhakti yoga and service with karma yoga. Many have attended her weekends where she may lecture and then proceed to give a loving embrace to a full line of seekers throughout the night. Many feel a deep sense of purpose, loving support and tremendous stream of kindness in her presence. I find it refreshing to have a woman who is energetically sharing the divine love presence and dispersing kindness, empathy, and service throughout the world.

I mentioned Swamiji Chidananda from Rishikesh and the Ramakrishna order of monks, Divine Light Society. I shared with you his saintly presence, his frail frame expressing with a dynamic voice, ways to know God. Inspiring stories from his childhood, his studies abroad in a Jesuit college, and the manner he includes and so knowledgeable on all religions. Humble, peaceful warrior for the Divine, no matter what religious belief you are sheltered in, yoga can enhance your prayer and meditation and give you greater insight upon your path. After all, aren't we all going home someday?

REACH AND RECEIVE: VALUE INTEGRITY

Find your teacher and path and feel safe, comfortable and with abundant enthusiasm for what you are a part of. Create integrity within yourself that is unbendable in this bendable yoga practice. Seek to be of assistance from your Sacred Heart and you will be serving from a stream of truth, love, and intelligence. Your aura will be seen and felt as a yoga teacher with good intentions to serve and create a better world for all.

Chapter 7

Waves and Whispers: Continuum

"You can't cross the sea merely by standing and staring at the water."

—Rabindranath Tagore

ONE EVENING, I was enlisted to pick up a well-known yoga teacher, Jean Couch, from the Cincinnati airport. CYTA was sponsoring a workshop the following day in 1985, featuring Jean and her Iyengar style of alignment teaching. She was the only Iyengar-style teacher who I admired, as she had such a sense of humor and lightness to this seemingly very rigid set of rules and cues when entering poses. Her book, *Runner's World Yoga Book*, was popular with athletes at that time.

I picked up this smiling, small-frame sprite of a yogi from the airport and drove her to meet other teachers for dinner at the now-extinct Alpha restaurant in the University of Cincinnati area. I believe there were five of us local teachers who enthusiastically greeted this California gem of a teacher to our city and yoga community. During the vibrant conversation of getting to know her, she made a comment about a teacher who she is currently studying with and a movement experience that deeply moved her in an unsettling yet curious way. "Unsettled", meaning not in a negative way, but rather, a deep longing to know and work with this new way of entering our bodies. She spoke of a particular technique, micromovement. The teacher of this and pioneering a new and deeper way of *exploring* movement rather than *doing* movement was Emilie Conrad Da'oud. The name of her work was Continuum. I listened while Jean shared her experiences with Emilie and Continuum Movement and how her enthusiasm for discovering a new way of being with movement had excited her.

Through the osmosis of deep listening and well, sitting beside her I suppose too, my curiosity was ignited to know and experience more about this "technique" and so I exclaimed, "Well, share this micromovement in the workshop!"

One of the teachers attending our soiree was an Iyengar teacher and brought to our attention the intent was an Iyengar-style workshop, which was sold out and that all participants were promised just that. Ah, but could we compromise in some way? Perhaps share the micromovement near the end of the workshop to give us a taste of what was authentic in Jean's study and teaching? Jean checked in with Emilie to see if she approved of her sharing. Well, it happened and thank goddess it did!

After a couple of days practicing Iyengar-style yoga, taking numerous notes, feeling stretched and stressed with the fullness of alignment, hours of standing poses with proper footage and torquing of hips, I was anxiously awaiting this last couple of hours of Jean introducing micromovement and Continuum to all of us.

Micromovement had interested Jean and ignited a newfound

passion of study and practice. Moments later, we all witnessed as she gave a few moments of demonstration what micromovement may appear to feel/look like. I recall being mesmerized by what I witnessed and aware also of others in the room who were distracted and somewhat disturbing with shuffling, sighing and a few whispers. I, however, was ready to dive in and explore! Ambient music by Michael Stearns accentuated the demo.

We were invited to lie down and relax as we yogis know how to do. Then as this interplanetary music which began softly gradually swelled, I felt the reverberation in my bones. My little finger began a simple movement leading me inward, my jaw so relaxed and the roof of my mouth felt expansive, and I recall gentle undulations from deep within my spine feeling as though I was floating on water. I was feeling the wholeness of my body as a deeply malleable organism! As this continued, my body felt like a delightful starburst of consciousness with millions of cells as stars freely floating throughout the universe while feeling supported with gravity.

Words are too structured to express this experience. I was in awe of the expansive nature of being starlight, a body of stars upon this planet. This experience seemed momentary, yet it had taken me on an inner journey that lasted over an hour. I recall hearing the voice of my best friend and yoga teacher extraordinaire, Jan Kolish, inviting me back to the room and reality. When my eyes opened, I saw Jan sitting beside me with a crystal pressing in my palm. Her smile, her voice and her presence enabled this cosmic starburst journey to root within my body as a cosmic adventure to share even now with you decades later!

I was surfacing slowly to earth with a heaviness felt in the body and with the tingling of being in total amazement. Jan acknowledged she was concerned as she witnessed me taking a deep dive into somewhere unknown without knowledge of where, why, and how to get her friend to return! I tried to put her at ease by teasing her placing of a lead crystal in my palm, not a quartz crystal. Though the lead probably did ground me to earth once again. Jan's love and best friendship would endure for another decade or so until her fateful return "home". A rare disease captured her lungs and after a lung transplant (she was one of first to receive back then) another year of slowing down to almost a crawl, she exited her body. Yoga brought us together in friendship and when it developed to a best friendship, I couldn't have been more blessed. I miss her presence to this. Daily morning phone calls, movies and Greek dance outings, trips, support for each other in so many ways, this was one of many gifts on yoga's pathway. Love is always a part of the journey.

In this same impactful workshop, I recall conversations with Jill McConnell, another amazing yoga teacher, who was studying to also become a massage therapist. She was not concerned as she witnessed my experience and with her smile and sparkling eyes, encouraged me to find out more. Jill had a vast array of study in many holistic modalities and saw how this micromovement experience drew me in to a new place. Her "seeing" was valuable and I honored her sharing of it with me.

The power of this day must be underscored, as I also met Vickie Fairchild, who was beginning her healing journey as an extraordinaire physical therapist, healer, and mystic. It was so admirable of her to come to a yoga teachers' event so wide open in her desire to learning more. Many years later, we would reunite sitting beside each other at a CYTA-sponsored dinner, I with a frozen shoulder and in need of therapy, and well, the rest is herstory! Vickie authored *The Divine Trilogy*, a mystical book titled that touched me to the core and inspired many moments of writing sacred experiences. We are the best of friends and continue this journey with love and enthusiasm while partying and celebrating enthusiastically too! Balanced in our being on earth.

Jean later told me she was amazed how I responded to the micromovement, going far within. She recommended I seek out learning and exploring more with Emilie herself.

I continued studying Continuum first with Jean at Omega Institute in New York. She did have a knowing understanding of this method of somatic movement and was a great friend and supporter of my continuing with Emilie and Susan. Jean also went another route studying *Balance*. She has created a tremendous study through her Balance Center in California, which I highly recommend. This work is beneficial for all students and teachers. Jean's style of teaching continues with intelligence, enthusiasm, and passion.

Needless to say, my foray into Continuum that day was a pivotal moment for my journey. Jean and I would see each other with her teaching expressions of Continuum at Omega Institute in New York and chose to experience the teaching from her, but knew, I was preparing for my main event, the deep dive into the new mystery with Emilie. I was on fire with curiosity of this profound work in consciousness explorations and found it to be all-consuming at times in my everyday life.

A book Jean suggested upon Emilie's recommendation was *The Mind of the Cells*, by Satprem. I went to the only new age bookstore in town, New World, and ordered. When I received, I recall circling, marking up lines on each page, which was so rich in its expression of what I felt I was just beginning to touch upon with these somatic movement experiences. I ended up ordering the entire thirteen-volume set of books/manuscripts of *Mother's Agenda* portraying the mother of Sri Aurobindo's ashram and teachings. These meditative experiences of the superhuman fed and nourished me in such a way of grounding the esoteric within my body. Rooting the experiences on earth rather than leaving the body during the practice of Continuum was also Emilie's teachings.

After a year or so, I penned a letter to Emilie, requesting she come to Cincinnati to facilitate a workshop on Continuum. She wrote back and knew of my great interest and experience through Jean, and said she was unable to come but her cofounder and teacher, Susan Harper, would be able to come. I was a bit disappointed but accepted the offer and contacted Susan. Susan would be such a delight to be with and had a commonality with Jean in the manner of which she seriously yet amusedly taught the depths of Continuum.

Susan would be a tremendous mentor for me on ways of sharing such deep, serious work but with humor and grace and lightness. She was the most sensual of teachers and unafraid to dive deeply wherever the waves moved her. This was exciting and inviting on so many levels! Susan happened to be married to the ambient musician Michael Stearns, whose music transported me to that heightened space Jan Kolish couldn't pull me from! Hearts of Space radio played Michael and his friends often. I would later visit their Los Angeles pad, meet Michael and attend a party, which included the author of *Medicine Woman*, Lynn Andrews. I was enthusiastically reading Lynn's shamanic series at this time, so what a bonus meetup!

Susan had a unique approach with Continuum and somatic studies. I was intrigued by her acute sensuality within the work and her encouragement to take this beyond walls and indoor workshops. Susan and Michael offered outdoor explorations for the deeper inward explorations. Their Green River trips in Utah and other landscapes were a new way to delve into the mysteries. After all, we are the inhabitants of earth and sky, we are the passion of molten lava and soft coolness of the moon. All dwells within us as the salt waters of oceans, the hum of the universe, the spirals of sacred dances and ancient chants, drumbeats that call the wild and pulse life through our veins. Continuum offered an array of ways to dive in and experience all our self. Not with a knowing of a subject to be taught and learned but rather, with a curiosity of the unknown mysteries, the creative force that whispers within the wind and waves of the river splash. Secrets to be discovered and known throughout our selves.

Omega Institute was the rustic setting for my initial meeting and study with Emilie. The trees, breeze, and heat formed a perfect setting for my wild, explorative introduction to Emilie, her shamanic tones, eye glances with long pauses of intent, which seemed to pierce through any obstacles of resistance to the whole experience. Her lectures would be the felt knowing also as her experiences she shared seemed to penetrate layers within one's psyche. Osmosis teaching would become a welcomed "familiar" the next few years with her.

After a couple of days listening and being in her presence, I phoned Jean on a payphone at the facility. I was delighted she answered my call, and I dramatically shared I was not impressed by Emilie at this moment and annoyed she lectured on and on… the work just didn't seem to feel the same. The word "same" would be significant context later, I would discover.

Jean asked what day of the retreat I was on. Day 2 of the five-day Continuum retreat. Her reply: "Oh, okay! On Day 3, you will feel the experience." I questioned that, but she encouraged me to stay, listen and feel.

This is a lesson around so many of the new teachings we take in. It takes a couple of days to unwind our expectations, our knowledge we bring in invisible file cabinets to open and unfold and to surrender to receive a new way of knowing, of exploring body, and trusting the wisdom within ourselves to jump off the cliff of what we know. Then we enter the spacious, new waves of learning.

Through this experience, I felt a swirling of being in a field of absolute virgin territory of knowing movement, the body, the interconnectedness with all of life. The rich textures in this somatic way of sensating my world was stunning. My hunger for learning and exploring only intensified. I was riding a current of curiosity. Well-supported through a new membrane of mystery, my intensity to know formulated ways to express and inspire a knowing that I share with my group of meditation students and yoga classes back home.

This was the beginning of a rewarding mentorship with both Emilie and Susan. I was onboard this train to a new destination and all in!

"All in" meant new terrain.

The deep dives of a ten-day retreat in the San Bernadino Mountains afforded a monumental jump off the cliff of knowing into an ancient and future abyss of the new! It took every ounce of courage I had to join with thirty others from around the world comprised of seekers of all faiths, paths, yogis, doctors, and scientists who had some prior touchpoint with Emilie, Susan, a taste somewhere in the world of Continuum, which left one hungry and thirsty for more.

As the retreat began, I walked up the narrow dirt path to my assigned cabin, noticing a woman with a confident smile and stride approaching me. Extending her hand, she said, "Hello, I'm Kate Jones from San Francisco, and whom might you be?"

This was the introduction to a lifelong, lovely supporting friendship that endures. As a sidenote, Kate's mother, Dorothy, just turned 101 years old and is a survivor from World War II who continues with Kate's assistance to be celebrated and acknowledged throughout the world.

From our first meeting at this Depth Retreat in Continuum, our friendship continues with rich conversations from the dimensions of a somatic knowing. Kate is a treasure in my life from our first meeting to present day. Movement creates deep relationships, too!

Emergence of New Waters: M'ocean

It felt so exhilarating to pull up in the van with other retreatants to the majestic Sky-High ranch nestled in the San Bernadino mountains, east of Los Angeles, for our ten-day Continuum retreat. Emilie walked out and greeted us. She invited us to check in and take our time to explore the epic scenery and grounds of this retreat place. Kate. my brand-new friend, and I, couldn't wait! We marveled at the cabins ahead and imagined what changes in ourselves awaited.

We gathered for a delicious dinner, then an evening gathering and introduction for the retreat. Both Emilie and Susan shared what the landscape for diving in might be structured like. For example, they expressed how during these longer endeavors of learning, participants come to an agreement to sharing in several consecutive days in silence, while all with sleeping bags in the central room. I had never heard of such a retreat experience of three days, twenty-four hours together, in a central room.

We agreed to the journey and which day it would commence. I had no idea how this would come to be but went along with the group in a unanimous agreement. The first few days were immersive, experiential moments of lectures followed by a practice dive. I would thoroughly feel nourished when each would speak of the "work" with their own resonance of Continuum. Each thought and expression felt like an ancient sound undulating through our mind-heart-body collective. Summoning the teacher within me, I took notes on ways to perhaps articulate how I would teach it. This new way of being in learning was pioneering a mystery from ancient and future knowledge. The two intertwine as a kundalini spirals up throughout the spine, full consciousness opening new landscapes for being and learning.

Emilie fascinated with her neurobiology knowledge, which stretched new avenues of consciousness to be seen, heard. Susan's sensuality of words touched the body into a relaxing response. Their balance in expressing Continuum was an impeccable somatic shamanic journey.

The courage to allow an unwinding and dissolving of what we came with, including our expertise in any field or previous ways of being human in the body, was immense throughout the group. These journey men and women were extraordinary in their own awakenings and our collective tribal experience. I so long for this once again! It was a breakthrough for all who attended and rippled out as earthquakes to affecting many other lives for the following years. When we share with our teaching a workshop, class, a conversation, a "seeing" moment, we continue this wave of wonder and beauty and unfold the wisdom of ages, both past and future, in the remarkable present moment of being.

I'll state it again: Yoga and somatic movement explorations are a marriage of the miraculous journey of experiencing the teaching of "thy will be done on earth, as it is in heaven!"

The emergence of the new waters, the fecundity of animated ascendence into new realms of being human and eventually plateauing where it felt tender, raw, and extraordinary, still moves me in new directions with the courage and deep dives into the unknown realms of consciousness. I am rooted through my yoga practice and am an evolutionary explorer through my somatic shamanic Continuum work. The two have become one for me. My practice is unified in its exploring with the yin/yang of mechanical/quantum—not separate but rather, intermingled in spiraling unfolding into my potential! Yoga and Continuum are the waves and whispers of insight, of love's body emerging. I so wish this depth and field of knowing for *you*!

I am forever grateful for Emilie's gift to mentor me personally and help me navigate through health issues, life issues and flourish. Her mentoring was an intimate connection with a teacher sharing with the most delicate touch of a newborn, yet the intensity of the dive into deeper waters within the sea of the self. During the immersion retreat, I had a private session with her. I told her I was interested in her shamanic experiences in Haiti where she lived and danced and explored for a few years. In these moments, with my lupus flaring raw, red patches on my face, Emilie got out her favorite rose water spray and began spritzing my face, then gave me the bottle. It was a personal moment that connected us in a deep way of friendship.

A year later, she offered me to teach a gig she was requested to teach at a local retreat center for the Jesuits in Cincinnati. The head of this center had been coming to me for private sessions in my unique blend of yoga and Continuum explorations, so he was familiar with both of us. I agreed to teach this ten-day international retreat and each day, check in with her regarding my experiences and that of others.

The unfolding of my teaching and resonance with somatic exploration beyond traditional yoga was in full display here at Jesuit Renewal Retreat Center. It was a full participation of people from around the world. Their trust in what I was sharing, which invited a leap from their stoic traditions into something new, was a testament in courage and curiosity! It was a profound ten days for all of us.

This trust, this nudging, support, and companionship, was my initiation into teaching a new way to embody somatic movement and yoga. I would continue to offer workshops nationally and internationally with this work, I titled it "Love's Body Emerging". People who had attended invited me to their cities to share the blend of yoga and Continuum. What a dream!

Emilie is a constant presence in my life with my work and I continue to be amazed in extraordinary experiences with her even though she passed on a few years ago. My recent excitement to explore the neurobiology of octopus was initiated years ago from her lectures of this species' intelligence and ability to regenerate. I feel Emilie's presence in dreams and one, the day I read of her death. I had looked her up to reach out and return to be with her and saw this shocking news. It devastated me. Shook me to my core. That evening, I had an amazing dreamtime connection with her. We continue—just not here together on a physical plane. At times, I tear up when I feel her formless spirit. I am so grateful for the immediate friendship and trust of Susan, who encouraged and invited me to inquire in new ways. Susan encouraged me to find a way to integrate my yoga and Continuum Movement rather than leave teaching yoga for Continuum, which I had shared with her.

I hope our paths cross again for deeper dives into the m'ocean. Susan's gifts are earthly treasures in an extraordinary universe. With the digital age, you can view both on YouTube in interviews. This is such a cherished way to relive their experiential lectures and brilliance.

The 1980s were such an unleashing of tribal tributaries taking me on a cosmic ride into shamanism of ancient cultures, Continuum's undulating waves and whispers of unknown waters, mentors of meaningful, honorable pathways into great mysteries. I am forever grateful and bow before each teacher, each written word and expressions of encouragement and support.

Emilie, Susan and Jean are three of the most valuable mentors and cheerleaders of organic somatic movement studies I could ever possibly wish for! The value of a daily yoga practice is immeasurable in its health benefits on so many levels. The rootedness so important for the body especially in this extremely yin culture we live daily. The magnificent spinal moves for the electrical current to unleash its power, the breath to carry the prana throughout the body and its energy field, the calming and alignment, which occur with a simple practice, are major healing gifts.

For years, this traditional yoga was my constant companion on my journey. I invite you to explore the deeper dives with a somatic exploration as well. You will find how it opens your field of knowing with a most exquisite curiosity. It may connect you with a source to ignite a new way of yoga and be a beneficial healing for you.

> ## REACH AND RECEIVE: OPENNESS AND SPACIOUSNESS
>
> Allow yourself to pause on your mat, and let go of all instructions on alignments, asanas, and breath techniques. Feel the most micro, subtlest of movements or breaths. Be willing to be curious. Be in a realm of deep sensating textures and seeing with an open attention rather than a set conclusion.

Note for Somatic Movement Students and Teachers

My dear deep travelers: I value the exquisite nature of these moments in movement. They offer a unique field of knowing and unfolding of consciousness, which ignites an enthusiastic curiosity for knowing more. We delve into a spacious m'ocean of experiences that move our understanding and conceptual knowing into a new place.

The blending of this with a traditional exploring of yoga helps to root this knowing and gives value to being in the body on the earth and grounding. The spinal moves and breathing techniques are a cosmic science of the ancients that has helped us evolve on this beautiful mother earth, our home.

There is deep value in the comingling of these two fields of knowing and I assure you it wasn't easy for me at first. But with others like my mentors in somatic movement encouraging me to explore a relationship with the two, I can honestly say to you, it is well-worth you exploring also a yoga practice with your somatic studies/explorations. Be curious and be balanced and be rooted in your miraculous body and let's unfold and witness Love's Body Emerging!

The All Love Yoga and Somatic School is not a brick-and-mortar structure but rather, an open field where we all can participate in evolving yoga and somatic movement studies. It is an opportunity for you to deepen the organic quality of your life and explore a new frontier for body and its connection and communication sensitivities. This current of evolution is exciting and the unfolding of Love's Body awaits all our participation.

The way of participating can be individual personal sessions, class sessions or in-depth dives of a retreat and play shop. You can also sponsor a group activity in your area and include a private session for yourself. The All Love Yoga and Somatic School is searching for inspired participants to carry on the deeper work and consider mentoring with us on your journey. If you feel a tug within your heart, a flutter of interest and enthusiasm, be in touch!

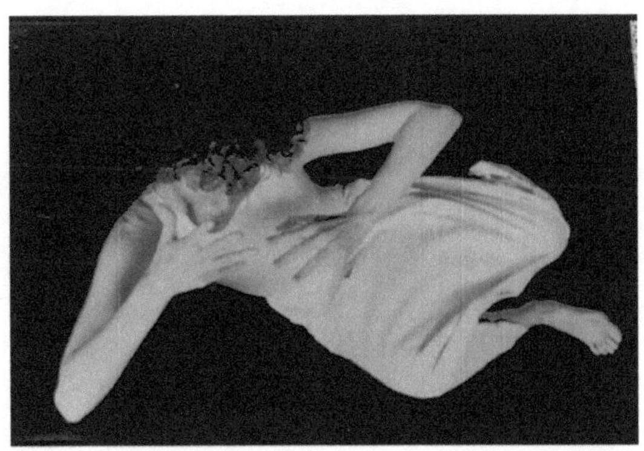

Continuum in practice. Photo by Alice Lambert.

Chapter 8

Language of the Drum
and Sacred Music

"After silence, that which comes nearest to expressing the inexpressible is music."

—Aldous Huxley

MY JOURNEY HAS been a tapestry woven of incredible experiences including multicultural meetings with masters of music and sound. Since childhood, as I have mentioned, I was enthralled in the Gregorian chants and loved singing the Latin versions of the Mass. The contemporary music and renderings of worship occurred while I was in high school and during the Vatican Council headed by Pope John XXIII.

Our high school invited a local priest who led a guitar mass celebration, one of the first in our area. It was cool with rhythms and lyrics, but the potency of a classic Gregorian chant is one of elevated energy. Probably similar in respect to classic Sanskrit and the powerful energy of certain mantras when recited on the yoga rosary, mala beads. Yoga and my Catholicism had similar ways to express prayer and meditation.

Early in childhood, my family had vacationed in the Great Smoky Mountains and visited a Cherokee Indian reservation. I was so excited to visit and explore this culture. I recall being focused on a particular Native American I referred to as "chief". He was playing a drum and I so wanted to dance! Later, I took a class in American Indian dance at a local park. It felt so familiar; the moves, the drumbeats seemed to return me somewhere.

Meeting Baba Olatunji

While studying with Jean Couch at Omega Institute, where a wide variety of programs are offered at the same time, I took my lunch break with a room full of others and would delight in hearing what they were studying. As I was engaged in conversation, a tap on my shoulder felt, I turned to see this beautiful African man with exotic robes requesting to sit beside me. Baba Olatunji, a renowned master African drummer, known to many drummers including Micky Hart of Grateful Dead and Sophie B. Hawkins. Well, the rest is history.

Baba was interested in hearing what I was studying, and I was interested in what he was sharing. "The Language of the Drum" was the title of his workshop and this language was studied throughout the world by master drummers and musicians! We had a break in our workshop that afternoon and he invited me to his "sampler" session. How could I resist? I told him of my interest in Native American shamanic drumming and my gifted purchase years before by a Taos Indian master drum maker, Red Shirt. This drum sits beside me now as a valued spiritual gift signed to me from Red Shirt.

"You will come and learn the language of the drum today," Baba said.

When Baba played the drum language you would imagine a presence so huge as he filled the space with his song and drumbeats. We were the same height, but I felt an immense stature whenever with him. I would return to Omega to study the drum even more with him, and then invited him to Cincinnati for a concert. The Cincinnati Zoo sponsored Baba and his entire group of drummers and dancers. It was a wild, humid evening in the summer. The performance exuded even more heat, dancing, chanting and lively celebration from a sold-out performance.

Baba and his troupe came afterward to my house for dinner and celebration. My students were angels helping prepare food and the house for their arrival. The house was bustling with energy, friends, students, and others attending this personal moment with the master drummer from Africa. A thunderstorm brewed and a few of his dancers in their traditional colorful African attire went out and danced to the beat of the rain and thunder, splashing in puddles on the sidewalks with radiant smiles.

I had been sharing in small groups in my home where I taught Continuum classes, private yoga and breathing sessions and some-times workshops. One was a drumming workshop where I shared the beat of our hearts, the beat of the different drums, and a lan-guage I had learned from Baba. He also loved to tease me from time to time. This moment he called me into the teaching space and asked me to share with him the language of the drum my stu-dents were sharing with him.

I was a bit timid but went ahead and shared the sounds of *gun go do pa* over and over with various rhythms. He laughed and enjoyed my moment of shyness. We had a love and respect for each other from the moment he tapped me on my shoulder. Baba also returned for another weekend workshop on African drumming of the language and the dance. The Contemporary Dance Theatre matriarch, Jefferson James, said yes to my request, and what a weekend ensued.

Baba and I had many phone conversations from his homebase in New York City. I also joined his workshop in New Mexico as it synchronized with my women's Chaco Canyon retreat. We all got to attend a Saturday with Baba and his group! I love the picture of us in that moment. Much later, I was crushed when I knew of his failing health and passing. The beat of his drum still resounds in my bone. "My dear African daddy", I would call him. What a gifted presence in my life.

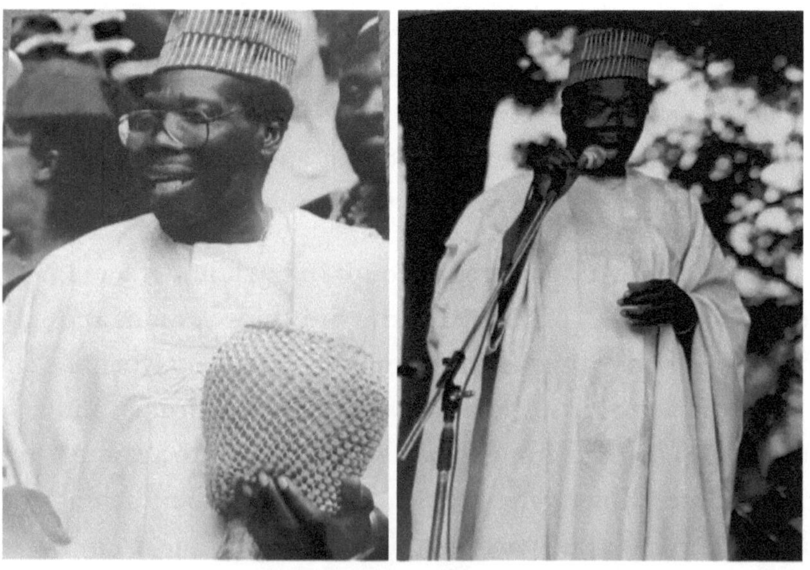

Beloved Baba Olatunji.

Yes to the Monks of Drepung Loseling Monastery!

Another request soon came from a healer in Indiana asking if I would be willing to sponsor Tibetan monks and their Sacred Dance Performance. She knew I sponsored many prominent people in yoga and other venues. I said yes as I always did. After my yes, she informed me it would be the end of December, in a few months, during Christmas week. How to pull this off for attendance, location, residency…oh my! But as my grandmother would say, "It'll all come out in the wash." Whatever that means.

I got busy, looking for a place for the venue, talked with University of Cincinnati and booked a hall for the event. Then where could I find rooms for ten Tibetan monks to stay? Ah, yes, the Jesuit Retreat Center, only a few blocks from my home. I called and they agreed to my delight. However, during Christmas week the staff who would have been there to cook meals would not be available.

Next door to the retreat center was a nursing facility, which I called on a whim, and they said yes for breakfast for the visiting Tibetan monks.

Covering my basics now to get the word out. I truly was doubtful if I could manage to cover any expenses during Christmas week and expected a low attendance. This took all the trust in manifesting I could muster up. And it happened! Sold out performance of their Sacred Music Performance during Christmas week. A local TV station also followed us around all week with great coverage and publicity.

Now I had no idea what to expect when an oversized van with a trailer attached pulled up in front of my house. Ten saffron robed monks stepped out one at a time and walked up the path to my front door. Chanting in a low tone, prayer hands, as they stepped into my home. What a sight!

We all sat around, sipping tea, with their manager helping with the language barrier different times. One of the young monks spoke fluent English and was helpful. A few yogi friends were there to greet and help, and I can tell you it is a meeting that lasts forever in your mind and heart!

One of the elder monks seemed distressed, awaiting a FedEx package from India. They had it addressed to my house. It was a form of chewing tobacco!

So here I was with ten Tibetan monks for a week, socializing and taking them to various events around town. One major event was with the Cincinnati Art Museum. I had asked if they would be interested in hosting a sacred sand painting by the monks. They also said yes! An unforgettable few days of the creation of the sand mandala, the ceremony of its disintegration, followed with a walk with the sand to a nearby water reservoir where they celebrated an ancient ritual of dissolving the mandala into the water. The museum told me that week they had more requests for memberships than ever before!

One fun experience with my monks was taking them to a Wendy's for lunch. This was in Milford, Ohio, a small community of mostly Christian followers. The monks felt hamburgers were the nearest to *yak* meat they were accustomed to in India and Tibet. We walked in and all ten monks pointed at the pictures above the cashier to what they wanted to eat. She rang it all up and while I was paying, my monks, all who were seated, broke out a low multi-toned chant. They pray for everyone, everywhere all the time. I looked around and not one person seemed to be bothered. It was as if I were the only one hearing this chant!

One of my monks ran off, and I saw him across the street going to the post office. He had a package to send. I am sure whoever was on the street in this quaint town that day had stories to share. I certainly do.

The monks would stay the day in my home, and their cook pulled out a giant pot and utensils the first day of the week for cooking meals during the day. I took him to Kroger to buy his staples. Now mind you, he spoke no English nor did I speak Tibetan. However, we communicated that I would drive him, walk him up and down the aisles so he could spot and load up any supplies. This was a fun time with him throughout the week. And on our kitchen stove, he stirred up great pots of soups, meats, and veggies. Still, after various performances they would ask me to take them to the "big boy place". They loved Frisch's Big Boy! Toward the end of the week, people were recognizing and acknowledging them after being featured on TV throughout their stay.

I had created a big event near Winter Solstice that week for my children's fund, a nonprofit I created upon my return from my adventure in Guatemala. I held many fundraisers with all proceeds going to various organizations, such as a shelter for women and children, an after-school program centered in downtown Cincinnati and an orphanage in Guatemala. The event this week of my monks visiting was extraordinary. With the assistance and creative direction of Betsy, a friend who I met to help with the organization, we created an evening vigil for displaced and abused children in the downtown area known as "The Banks". Toyota became a major sponsor and donated funds to make this happen.

The Tibetan monks were part of this sharing a performance with their Sacred Music. Dennis Banks, a known Lakota Indian also contributed with drumming, local women's choir, Muse, lending their beautiful harmonies were all part of the spectacular event. It was frigid, near zero degrees, but the monks' bare arms were unaffected by the stinging cold perhaps because of their Himalayan DNA. City council designated this day for the children local and around the world and presented the designation to me. What a monumental evening as the monks' bright orange/saffron robes stood out in the darkness of night among the crowd. God bless all the children of the world.

The Rinpoche ("Precious Jewel") gifted me with a mala bead and an envelope of the sand mandala and a prayer shawl. I value these precious gifts. My heart deepened and widened by their presence. Love my monks and their special sacred music they brought into my life! Multi-tonal chanting still resounds within my bones.

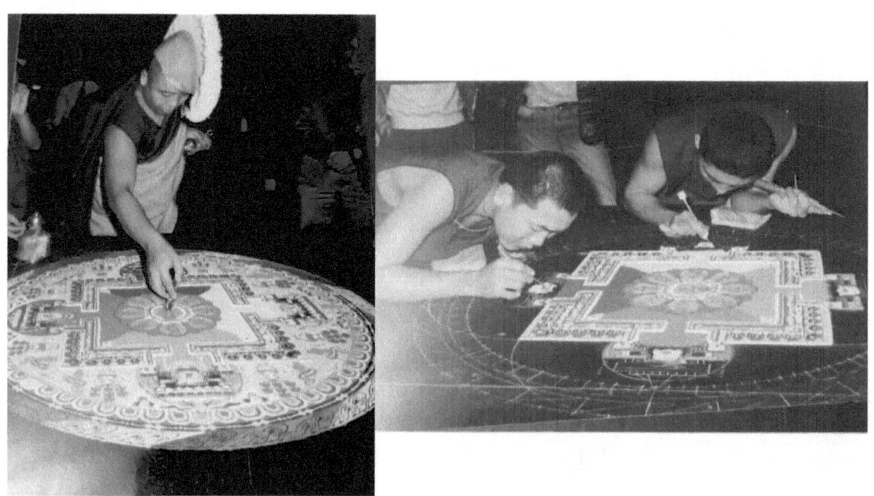

The memorable Monks of Drepung Loseling Monastery.

Here with Ram Dass

My experience for creating well-attended, interesting, and multi-cultural events in Cincinnati was spreading into diverse areas for presentations. I received yet another call from a gentleman, who was the manager for the iconic yogi and author of the seminal book, *Be Here Now*, Ram Dass. He was on tour throughout the country and again I said yes! This group was a well-oiled machine. They had their organizational skills fine-tuned and were a delight to work together on this event.

Again, I leaned on University of Cincinnati, renting Kresge Auditorium for a lecture by this prominent figure known to many since the 1970s. Back then, I attended a taping at the PBS studios when Ram Dass was a guest on Lilias's TV show. I recall listening as he offered a meditation visual for understanding the process. I use this visual today in workshops and retreats and value greatly being with him that day. Twenty years later, here I oversaw his visit! Life's gifts and wonders.

It was so easy to get the word out and have my living room buzzing with volunteers for this event. Each one was assigned a task from the ambiance of his hotel room, placing flowers, to selling tickets around the city, and monitoring guest lists and seating arrangements. The auditorium filled with people from the tristate area. I was honored to be on stage and introducing Ram Dass to the audience. His talk and Q & A afterwards electrified the new age audience as only he could do. This also was a fundraiser for my children's fund. I informed his manager from the first call I would graciously accept this task of sponsoring his appearance in exchange for the fundraising component.

It was a whirlwind of picking up at the airport, taking to the hotel, dinner and the event and gone next day. I couldn't have managed all this without the amazing support from yogi volunteers and from his manager, Dave, an expert at organizing such programs.

Later, Ram Dass suffered a stroke, and lived for some time after. We were blessed with his presence that magical evening.

When I reflect on the programs I created and offered in Cincinnati, I truly hope someone picks up this torch of possibilities and creates the variety of global offerings that are readily available. Imagine, this was all done without computers! These programs were a joy, a lot of work, and opened my heart to the service in yoga.

Within the yoga evolutionary journey of my body-mind-heart-spirit, I have been moved in other ways, inspired moments, sparks of energy which directed me in a new tributary of timeless learning and being.

These stories I am guided to share are rooted in my awakening of courage and confidence with yoga, Continuum Movement, and people and places along the way. Their inspirations mostly from my intuition unfurling its petals of possibilities into the unknown and with many nudges to go and explore, do and see, from others in my life. So often we receive these glimpses of other realities and possibilities but brush them away as a meaningless daydream.

I am sure I have countless moments of brushing away, but more true to my soul's journey, there are special, undeniable awakenings that turned into adventures. I offer them to you as encouragement to listen, to see, to dive into those daydreams with a conscious intention to learn what they may have to offer this life within your journey. With courage and confidence, let the impossible become possible, the ordinary become extraordinary!

REACH AND RECEIVE: INSPIRATION

Take a moment, feel into what or who truly inspires you and reach for it/them today. Allow the extraordinary of what you don't know to unfold its beauty and enrich your life today.

Chapter 9

Journey into Mayan Mysteries

*"And if a person is religious, I think it's good, it helps you a bit.
But if you're not, at least you can have the sense that there is a
condition inside you which looks at the stars with amazement
and awe."*

—MAYA ANGELOU

EARLY 1990, I was swimming in depths of my unfolding into unknown territories with a confidence and courage from both my rooted yoga practices and Continuum Movement deep dives. Practicing and teaching was inspiring and facilitated a comfort of the familiar, which nestled my consciousness with each workshop, class or individual session into a routine of weekly sessions. Predictability was present, yet within each session with another, I was so inspired by their quickening and deepening of awareness and healings. Today, I get goosebumps and tearful eyes when witnessing even on Zoom when participants are aligned and awakening.

As always in my journey with yoga and Continuum, I felt I

reached a plateau which was so comfortable, only to have a new door appear, an invitation to see and be more! Hesitation and excuses were tried in the beginning, but eventually the adventure appeared with all its unmarkable, unimaginable pathways to a new depth, a new unfolding. Shaking in my boots, so to speak, I could not refuse the adventure. It was shaking me with a soul's energy and purpose I could not pass over, brush over.

I was attending a gathering of holistic teachers in one of the known architectural wonders in Cincinnati. This massive stone structure was owned and shared by a woman who was a catalyst in bringing together many of us from a variety of modalities and experiences occasionally.

I enjoyed meeting friends and making new ones. On this evening, I met a young woman who shared her recent backpacking adventure to Guatemala. I listened and with a wonder around the thought of going alone to an unknown country and backpacking. I couldn't imagine, yet I was taking women out on adventures camping in the Southwest, Chaco Canyon, New Mexico. That was the most daring I have experienced. I shared with her these adventures of my own within the canyons, petroglyph trails, architectural wonders from another era where tribes gathered.

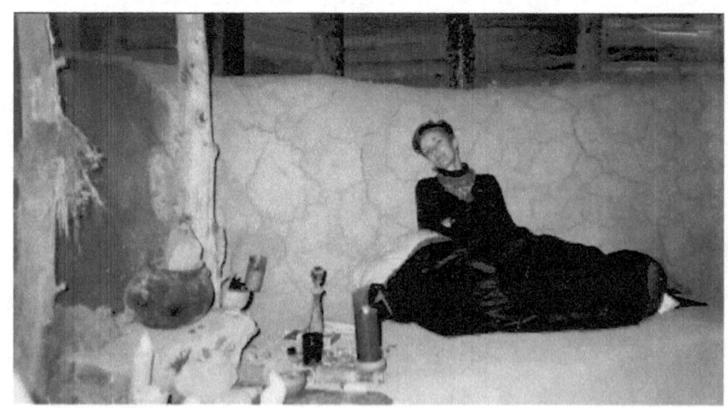

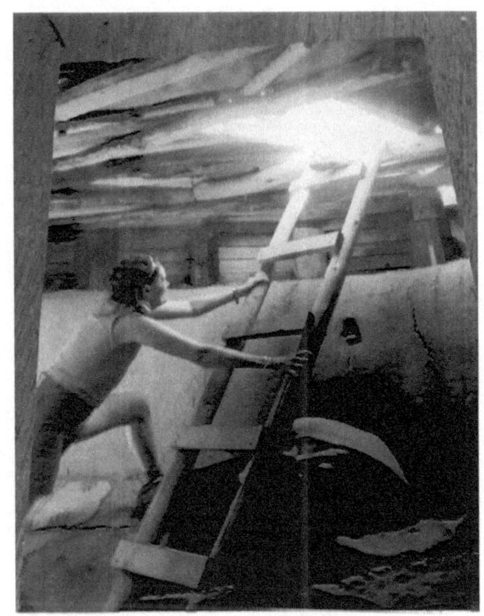

Kiva meditation and prayers ritual.

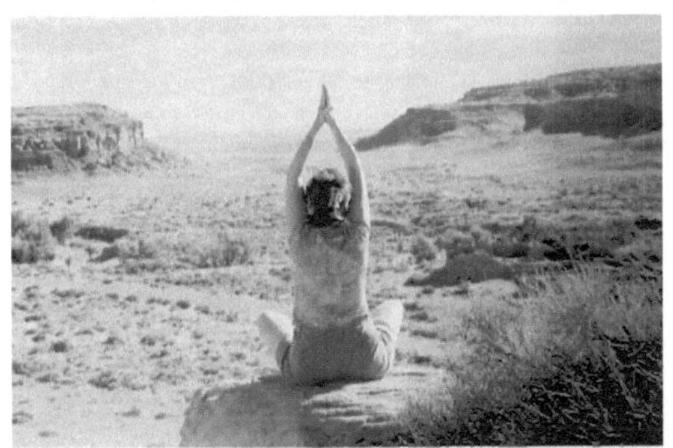

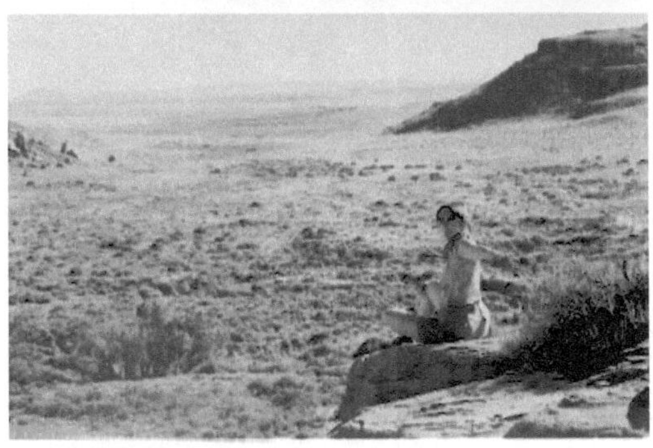

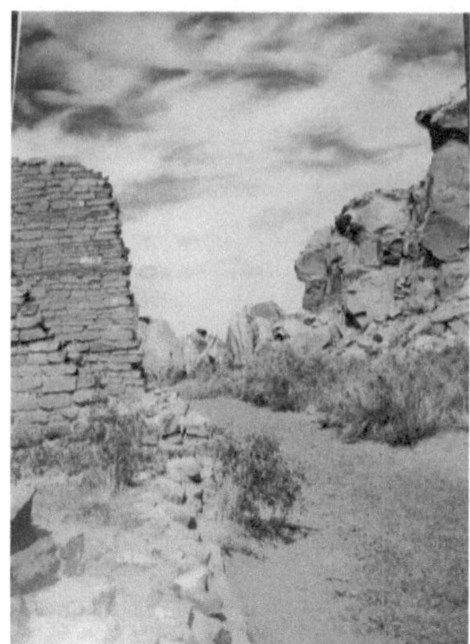
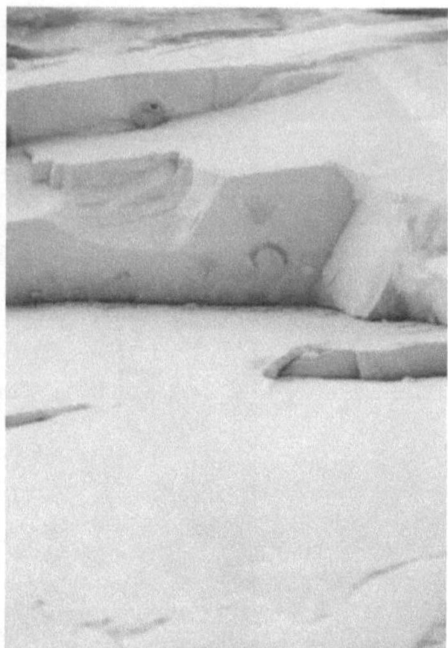
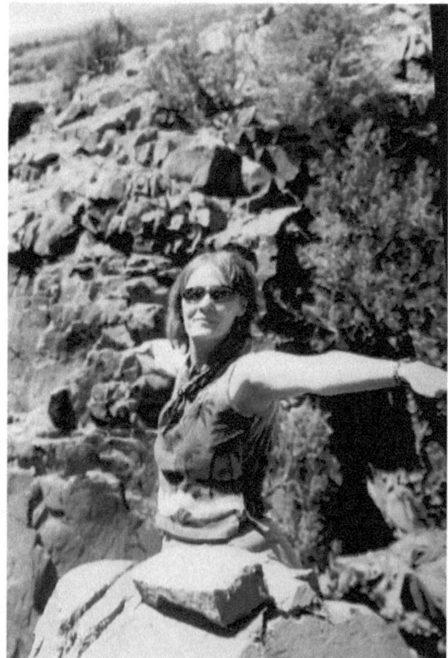

Women's Southwest Retreats in Chaco Canyon, New Mexico.

As I drove home, satisfied from great food, drink and conversation, this adventurous backpacking to Guatemala interested me a great deal. Our initial conversation was sparked by me noticing the rainbow colors of her vest, hat, and jewelry, which seemed to accessorize her story of Guatemala and backpacking. I am embarrassed to say, I didn't even know exactly where this country was in relation to Mexico.

As I shared my learnings with others throughout next few days, I noticed a visual of the rainbow colors and woven textures the Guatemalan backpacker wore would pop up in my mind's eye. At first, I thought maybe I simply needed more color in my wardrobe! Then I realized it felt like a deeper pulsation to *see*.

A few days later, I received a call from my friend, Suzie, who had a lovely eighty-acre farm nearby and was another catalyst in bringing together many seekers in the new age for learning and community, retreats, and programs with a wide variety of holistic and spiritual experiences. She invited me to attend a presentation of the Mayan culture. Still not connecting dots, I agreed.

We were all sitting out on the layered wooden deck adjacent to this remarkable century-old farmhouse on a Spring late afternoon, feeling the delicious sun's warmth melt away layers of cold from winter's wrath, daydreaming of summers past on this veranda with family and friends. Power lounging with a quenching thirst and soothing hibiscus tea in hand now, so many years later, I recall celebrations, studies and teaching here over the years.

I listened to the woman's talk about the Mayan and their culture with interest but honestly felt her presentation to be somewhat dry and it took little more energy to listen, pay attention than usual. My daydreaming was quite active. When she mentioned Guatemala, I perked up. Again, the vibrant rainbow colors appeared in my mind's eye. Interestingly enough, the sun's angle created a filtered rainbow of light upon the deck this very moment. Enough so, it blurred the view of the speaker momentarily. This caught my attention and felt a pulling in a direction. A "wake up and see and listen" moment! I let this slip away too. As she ended the first part of her program and took a break for the second part, which included a slide show, I felt I wanted to slip out the door, drive down the winding, gravelly farm road home.

I was saying my goodbyes when the speaker approached me. I thanked her and said I needed to go but did share with her the moment of rainbow color memories and the sun and Guatemala. I mentioned I was going to seek more information and thanked her for her presentation. She paused and looked me in the eyes, touched my arm and said, "Diana, I feel you might want to stay for a few moments longer and view the slides. I feel moved to say this to you."

I did not want to disrespect her intuition. To be polite, I said I would. I sighed inside because I really wanted to go on a nice, sunny day's hike at the nature center nearby! I proceeded to the darkness of the den and sat with others on the floor for her slide presentation.

Shades and curtains were pulled to darken the sunlit room. I sighed, feeling a missed opportunity to hike in the sunlight. After a few comments, the slideshow began. She was sharing her trip to various Mayan sites in Guatemala and in Yucatan, Mexico. From the first slide to the last, I was transported with a current of consciousness in which these sites felt so familiar, holy, home, recognizable with sight and feelings that were overwhelming. I had tears streaming down my face and tried to wipe them away as I would brush away a daydream. I felt my nervous system quaking as though an unleashed wild energy was released throughout my body and containing it was laborious. I had no words for this experience. I had tremendous feelings of longing to return home.

I sat there in shock. Awed by what I experienced, I am even now reliving this as I write and share with you, with tears filling my eyes so they are blurred. Blurred as the sunlight that day on the deck. This was a moment of waking up and threading the Mayan colors for a future adventure to return home by returning to an unfamiliar or known place within myself.

The lecturer noticed and smiled. I am grateful for her intuitive knowing in that moment and shared this with her. All these occurrences were within a week's timeframe. Is it surprising the following morning, I received a call from a friend out west who shared she was going to Guatemala in July to study Spanish in Antigua? Of course not! After sharing with her my experience, I was encouraged to obtain a passport and meet her there. We could backpack throughout the country together. *Whew!* I took a deep breath and that very day, went to the post office, and applied for a passport with a "rush" on its arrival. Follow through on a daydream!

The following few months, I began the preparation for this journey with a checklist. Inquiring what a backpacker in Guatemala might need as far as clothing, and, of course, a backpack including items such as rainsuit, mosquito netting, the attire from head to toe included good hiking boots, hat, long pants with many pockets, Swiss army knife set, light-weight clothing, towel/wash cloth, bandanas, canteen (before fashionable water bottles), collapsible dish set, an air mattress, and malaria pills.

The required shots and security briefs from the state department did have me wondering from time to time what the heck I was in for. Nonetheless, knowing my friend was going to be there was a safeguard I needed to continue on the track of preparing for a July trip to Guatemala. Each day, I would place my backpack on my shoulders and walk throughout my neighborhood, then placed a brick in it, increasing the weight.

I studied conversational Spanish to get by on, hoping I would be able to retrieve and optimize my two years' worth of high school Spanish classes. Wish I had paid more attention to verb conjugation, darn it! But my passport arrived in plenty of time for this journey. My friend, Alice, a photographer, briefed me on the art of capturing through the camera lens my adventure and with her Native American path of experience/study. She provided a block of film (no digital at this time). I had a good Canon camera to practice the art of seeing. This was an important part of my journey as it enabled me to chronicle the places I would experience with expansive seeing and feeling and a rich array of Mayan memories to enjoy to this day, decades later.

The day arrived to fly out of Cincinnati and after a layover, fly into Guatemala. I recall two distinct things about this arrival. I was exhausted, most likely from no sleep from anxiety the night before, and the stench of urine as I walked through a tunnel to airport baggage claim. I recall picking up my backpack and feeling the force of its weight. wondering how on earth I would be able to hike with it for a few weeks!

I do remember being impressed with the clouds of black exhaust from old Blue Bird school buses from up north, puffing out into the air. My friend, Annie, suggested I cover my mouth and nose with a bandana. When I did, I was surprised to see black gunk expelled from my sinuses when blowing my nose. *Yuck!*

We stayed in the city a couple of days so I would acclimate to the climate of weather and culture. I walked around, hearing and seeing the sounds and sights of another land on this earth. It felt both foreign and familiar in an odd way. I so wanted to fluently speak Spanish or one of many dialects of Mayan language spoken throughout Guatemala. But I was only able to speak the basic, ordering eggs, bread, and coffee and of course, *galletos* (i.e. cookies)! (I made certain I knew that translation.) Instant coffee served in a bowl was a real coffee lover's worst experience, but days go by, and one acclimates to even this tasteless drink. I also carried liquid oxygen to drop thirty droplets in a gallon of water to help kill anaerobic bacteria. An acquired taste but necessary. Purchasing sheets of toilet paper in public restrooms was also a new experience. Children sold these items as income for their families.

Just as I got used to the city, we were off on a crowded school bus westward to Panajachel. The winding hillsides were scary. But viewing the terraced landscapes and gardens alongside the rainbow attire of Mayan was so exhilarating. It helped dissipate my fear of the treacherous ride with these beautiful cliffside views. Chickens were passengers on villagers' laps, cackling throughout the steamy hot ride to Panajachel. Then you had daring people atop the bus holding on for the fast, winding ride. I cannot imagine ever volunteering for that bus pass!

Once we arrived safely, I let out a huge sigh and laughter from this very original excursion. Sifting through my backpack after we got away from the dispersing crowd of people and animals, I was astounded to find my camera missing. I couldn't wrap my foggy head around how someone could have snatched it. But then again, I had been preoccupied with survival! The thief must have sensed it, too. Here, I could have allowed internal chaos to set the stage for this important trip, but I summoned calming thoughts. Someone would be making good use of that Canon.

We walked through the small village of Panajachel onto a dirt road to then hike to a friend of a friend's place where we were welcomed to stay for two nights. The owner was out of town on business and her little house in the outskirts of the village was cared for by a local Mayan couple and their two children. They were so kind and welcoming and were serving us graciously with a cold bucket of water to shower, literally a bucket which you pulled the rope and rinsed off with. We bought a few items of vegetables, rice, snacks and enjoyed a hot meal "at home".

Candlelight provided the light in the evening, as there was no electricity. It was a soothing alternative to lights and a way to align with the rhythm of the evening hours. Annie and I were both journal writers, so we had our personal quiet time to do so. Sleeping in a bed was to be a luxury as I would soon find out. Up early with sunrise piercing through the window, we ventured out to the lake and took a boat across to Santiago. I marveled at elderly, small-framed women carrying a load of logs upon their backs and other items like baskets of flowers upon their heads. Men carrying sewing machines on their heads into town to tailor garments. An unbelievable demonstration of physical strength everywhere. All were attired in the rainbow colors of the Mayan people. Their smiles and open-heart greetings were so touching and impressive.

We wandered through the village market, ate breakfast at an open-air café, bought sundries at the marketplace such as jade figures, a wooden mask, and flowers for the housekeeper. As we walked through the village and visited churches along the way, children approached us in hopes of selling bracelets and jewelry. I would buy one item from each child at first and sometimes asked if I could photograph. The pictures hang upon my walls to this day. Beautiful memories and radiant smiles of the Mayan people.

When we returned to Guatemala City the next morning, I felt

a restlessness and realized a few things. I was adventurous, but I was following Annie's lead everywhere. She would talk Spanish, figure out bus schedules and locations, places to eat, etc. This was the first week of being in Guatemala and something was brewing. I could feel it pulse, making me uncomfortable.

Upon arriving in Guatemala, Annie and I had decided after sharing some experiences with each other, we would part ways. I was uncertain if I could manage traveling alone and after an evening of consideration, decided to make some calls the next day. Off to the local phone location, where you waited to use a pay phone. I called two people that day. First, my therapist, who was so reassuring that whatever I decided it would all be fine. But I sensed she would feel more comfortable if I returned to Cincinnati. My next call was to my friend, Alice, who encouraged me with her voice and directive coming from her belly, to go to the town center, purchase a few slide disposable cameras, and return to the village to stay in the house another night so I could feel into my next stop on the journey.

Alice's encouragement was the push I needed, and I took her advice. Needing directions and food, I drew upon my high school Spanish and the little book I had of translation to help. I did it! On to the bus and return to the village of Panajachel on my own.

I arrived and found the housekeeper surprised by my return. I tried to explain "Only one night…friend elsewhere…need to plan my continued journey." It was confusing but we agreed somehow this would work out. She and I sat at the candlelit table, pointing at objects and exchanging Spanish terms. She would then speak her native language, Katchigal, and I would say it in English. This went on for a while. It was such an impressive moment in my life. Here I was from a suburb in Cincinnati, now in a village in

Guatemala, sitting at a table with a Mayan woman sharing our stories as best as we could.

One moment, she paused and with little Spanish, gestured beneath her eyes and said, "Tu es triste?" *Are you sad?*

It touched my heart, and I put my hand upon my heart and acknowledged, "Si." I mostly felt anxious and unaware of what I was doing there at all. I thanked her for her time and sincere conversation of getting to know each other. I prepared to sleep in the bed still contemplating my purpose. I had little sleep, as I was disturbed by what I heard through the night I thought were fireworks coming from across Lake Atitlan. Maybe a celebration. This would be important later during my trip. I finally fell into a dreamy sleep and woke with the morning rays warming the room. I showered with the provided bucket of water, tried to unload items from my backpack to make it lighter, and offered them to the family.

After warm hugs and radiant smiles, I set off into my future. With a spirited stop at a market stand, I went to the shore of Lake Atitlan and three young girls approached me as I sat meditating. I asked their names. We spoke briefly and they wanted me to take their photo, which I have framed in my creative space today. I bought a few bracelets from them. Their youthfulness lifted my spirits. I made a plan to return to Guatemala City for the night and onto Tikal, the famous ancient Mayan capital city. My stride now was confident, and with the backpack from hell on my shoulders, I continued my journey alone and curious.

Finding a seat in this stinky, crowded, old Blue Bird school bus was challenging. In between people racing to sit, people climbing to sit atop on roof with luggage, I found an open seat next to an elderly Mayan woman. I recall the wrinkled, timeless face and felt how beautiful! I wondered what stories each wrinkle in time could share. The heat already showed up on our perspiring faces, which we wiped with bandanas, treasuring a small bottle of water used for pouring relief onto it and sipping. We were off with the jerky, manual-shift drive through the narrow, mountainous paths, loud talking, babies crying, chickens cackling. I fantasized about a bath and bed in the main city.

The terraced gardens and rainbow dresses on the side of mountains breezed past. When the bus flew downhill so it would have steam to get up the next hill, my Catholic prayers appeared in my mind. "Remember, oh most gracious Virgin Mary, that never was it known that anyone who fled to thy protection, implored thy help or sought thy intercession, was left unaided…!" One of my favorite prayers I would recite at night with my little altar behind my bed, a statue of the Sacred Heart of Mary, which comforted and soothed me to my core.

Those bus rides were frightening enough and when you saw the many white crosses with flowers where accidents occurred, well, one would gulp in fear. As if the bus ride itself didn't bring enough anxiety, we came to a halt suddenly. The tone of conversation intensified. The bus driver opened the door. This was not unusual stopping here and there to pick someone up. But the tension in the bus was palpable. A man with a gun boarded, speaking in a demanding tone toward the bus driver and peered down the aisle. The driver got off the bus and to my surprise, all the men on the bus were escorted out and lined up against the bus. Heart racing, sitting against the window with a full view of the activity, I discretely pulled out the disposable camera from my daypack and began to click the scene in frames. This is one of my slide presentation's more dramatic pictures. I noticed a USA stamp on the guns. Weeks later, when I arrived home, I would go to the library in Cincinnati and look for books on the history of Guatemala. I learned that the "fireworks" I heard at night was gunfire. I had no idea of the political turmoil and civil war transpiring amidst my spiritual journey.

At this moment, however, I was calculating how I would fight to survive. I moved from my seat to an aisle seat, staring up to the front where the gear shift was in full view. If I heard one act of violence or shot, I planned to book it up the aisle and throw the bus in gear as it was still running and take off! It was a robbery. All the men had to give their money to the wildly younger men with guns. There was no violence, thank goodness, and the driver was first to get back on board, with the passengers following. The gunmen took off into the field probably to await another bus. One of my photos captured a young man staring right into my camera. It reminds me of this chilling moment and never once after did I complain about the bus ride itself being scary. I was happy to fly down those hills and get to the city!

After respite at a hotel and the luxury of a bed and restaurant, where I lightened my load figuratively and mentally for two days, I boarded yet another bus on a two-day journey to Tikal. On the final stretch to Flores, I met a lovely newlywed couple from San Francisco who were there on their honeymoon. We shared our adventures we experienced thus far and bonded. We exchanged information and when home, months later, I was in San Francisco teaching a workshop on movement with my friend, Kate. She had booked me also in a local college to give a slide presentation on my Guatemala journey. The couple attended, and it was so remarkable to share our stories together with the group.

Stopping in Flores, to sleep in a hammock in a room in

a hostel, I'm not sure I could have done this without my new friends. They were a support and friendly companions during this part of the adventure. Over my hammock I stretched out the mosquito netting I was still carrying because it was the lightest item in my backpack. I placed my boots beside it and hoped to rest. Mosquitos were buzzing and annoying, so I was restless in my leisure. I tried to turn over on my side and oh no! A scorpion strutting across the floor. How could something so small rule the room? But it did. I now sat up in my hammock and wondered what to do and if there were extended scorpion families observing me from their hiding places! I watched it intently through sleepy eyes as it turned and began a route toward my hiking boots. Well, in yoga, we practice ahimsa, non-violence toward all creatures. I am known to gather spiders, flies, insects and gently carry them outdoors back home. But this?

I exclaimed "Ahimsa!" as I sent him off into another realm. I still wear these boots for gardening at home. And think about a small creature that lost its life on the sole of my boot. For an empath, this is troublesome.

I managed to get a few hours of fragmented sleep in before packing up and exiting in the morning. I had a nice breakfast at the open-door café with my new San Fran friends, sharing our sleepless-night adventures starring mosquitos and the scorpion. We then boarded yet another bus to take us into the ancient city of Tikal. During this entire trip, I felt the presence of people I met from around the world in occasional moments I was doubting my ability to continue or feeling intense sensations of loneliness. My angels were present and caring during this adventure.

Once we entered the national park, I bought a map of the city so I could navigate the paths to the Mayan temples and ruins. We walked to the area where overnight hammocks were available. I chose one, set up my backpack and began putting items into my day pack for my first excursion into this ancient landscape that had been calling me for months. Taking in the magnitude of it all, I observed the many tourists juxtaposed with the incredible structures. I was so proud of myself for arriving in this place and pushing through fear and uncertainty. I was ready!

The morning heat and humidity crept in and thickened the air I breathed. As I walked toward the center plaza, I felt deep focus and gratitude for walking on an ancient path created by peoples of eons ago in a then vibrant culture and city. Were they still here in spirit form? I heard a faint call from someone. Oh, someone actually answering my question? It became louder. "Diana!" I turned quickly and there in the distance, I saw my friend, Annie. What an unexpected reunion after two weeks!

We shared our stories and then made a pact to finish out this last week of our stay together. We explored the ruins, meditated in these ancient structures, and studied their history in the evenings while lying on our hammocks. We walked the dirt paths to the Temple of the Inscriptions, and I sat upon a crumbling, sandy stone wall to journal. Journaling my thoughts, revelations there in the temple where ancient writers inscribed history and the *Popul Vuh*, a text recounting the mythology and history of the K'iche' people of Guatemala. I tore pages of blank paper from my journal and rubbed dirt over carvings. I placed them back into my pages to keep forever.

Annie and I explored various sites and got caught in heavy afternoon downpours. One afternoon, we befriended two young gentlemen from Germany, and they joined our late afternoon excursion to denser area and to Temple #4. Out of sight, we climbed the unexcavated structure, grabbing onto vines and stones, and made our way to the top. We entered the doorway to a dank stone enclosure and decided to spend the night high above the rainforest and in the temple. Quite an experience I would not have embarked on without the security of others and these kind gentlemen who were explorers as well.

Dusk fell upon the rainforest. We heard a ranger calling out for anyone there and didn't answer. We became one with the evening of the rainforest as monkeys and toucans screeched through the night. It was a full moon as well! We sat on the temple's edge. It was creepy at first but then the vista of treetops looked like a velvet green carpet as far as the eye could see. Tops of the famous temples in the plaza lifted above. I had a crystal ball, which we took turns with holding up to our eyes and looking through to the full moon that lit up our faces and smiles. They spoke English and that was good since we spoke no German. All four of us were in awe that we were experiencing this magical evening! We chanted, meditated, laughed. In some moments, tears streamed from the power of our meeting and being here together.

At one point. I found myself on the side upon a ledge feeling a sense of ritual, of Sacred Source the Mayans must have felt and known. It was a powerful moment of healing, of reaching and receiving from another culture in this present day. I was now sobbing though not sure why, I felt I had returned home. I gave thanks in my own little ritual, leaving a crystal upon the top of the temple.

We crept carefully off the ledge into the doorway at the top of the temple, checking our surroundings, laid out our sleeping bags, crawled in and bid a good eve to each other. Deep gratitude was overwhelming as I laid there amazed at where I was! The pictures I have matted and framed still carry my attention back to this moment in my life. The picture being atop this temple and looking out over the rainforest toward the main plaza where the well-known Jaguar temple towers high above the lush forest is one of my favorites.

We all woke up startled by a rash from head to toe though Annie had somehow been spared. I was also intensely nauseated, and after our morning descent down the stone and vines, which was scarier than the ascent the day before, we parted ways. Annie and I returned to the hammocks. All the way, I would have to walk into the thickness of plants off the path and get sick. I was dehydrated for sure after this day and could not eat for a day or so.

Like it or not, bus time again.

Another village to board a small boat to take us on a river trip to Mexico. What could possibly go wrong? Of course, the boat person took us to an unscheduled stop where we were asked for our passports and would have to "donate" money to continue on our journey. Frustrating but we were able to escape and be on our way to Mexico. We slept overnight in the first village, sleeping in our hammocks outdoors of a hostel/café. I have beautiful photographs of a family who ran out on the dirt path to greet me when I strolled on into the small town in search of water and food supplies. We continued our journey with many bus rides around the Yucatan peninsula, exploring Loltun Cave and the shamans' markings on walls, to Palenque atop the Temple of the Crone and Uxmal, where we hung in the circles of the infamous ball court. We hiked through rainforest to a magnificent waterfall where we parted ways for a few hours to explore, journal and soak up the beauty in our own way.

I sat above the waterfall camouflaged and observed others hiking and approaching. I was there for a couple hours and so interested in noticing various responses to receiving the experience. I journaled about the "seeing". Then while alongside the unexcavated Temple of the Crone, I sang "Hotel California" for some bizarre reason.

A *final* bus to Mexico City and we flew off to our respective homes. A journey of a lifetime. My fortieth year on earth initiated with vast adventure and unsurpassed beauty. With my yoga, meditation, and Continuum Movement studies, I am certain I could not have imagined anything remotely close to this journey for myself.

My arrival home took some time to acclimate being in a city and into a routine once again. The dishwasher, washing machine and dryer seemed like luxurious and unnecessary items in my home. I would be interviewed about this adventure and written about in the *New Lifestyle Magazine*.

I went downtown to the main library and gathered books to read about Guatemala and its history, as well as its magical Mayan culture. I found out about turmoil and its history. I read about the Mayan woman, Rigoberto Manchu, whose tale of survival in this turmoil was remarkable.

Being in Guatemala, backpacking and exploring was an initiation into a new depth of courage and confidence for sure! But also, the lingering rainbow presence draws my psyche back into another time.

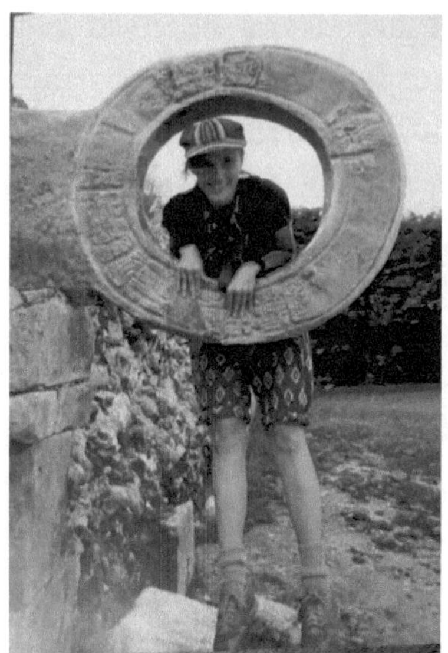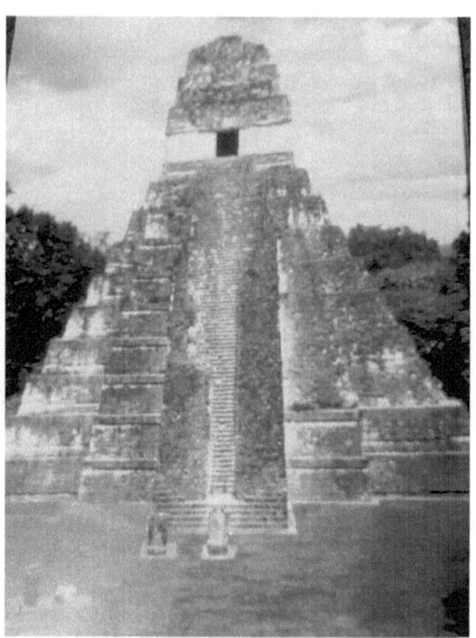

Guatemala and Uxmal, Mexico journey.

REACH AND RECEIVE: ADVENTURE

What adventures have captivated your attention? Have you taken your yoga and somatic movement practice out beyond walls of your home or studio? Have you created moments to be connected with ancient times to present? What is the wildness within you seeking adventurous expression? The untamed, unusual, unnamed is swirling with possibility. Feel and see the everyday ordinary become extraordinary. Go…have your adventure!

Chapter 10

Magical Lands and Waters

"Wilderness is not a luxury but a necessity of the human spirit."

—EDWARD ABBEY

SOMETIMES THE RAINBOW presence reminds me of a more recent past than a foreign yet familiar period like my adventure in Guatemala. At times, you "know" when you've been somewhere before. And it may not be the physical place itself. The reminder may be to reflect on a milestone and your evolution. Reflection is recognition; recognition of the obstacles you overcame or bravely traveling thousands of miles away from an old comfort zone. Reach and receive your growth! To underscore this explicit need for reflection—and the satisfaction of realizing how resilient you are—I've chosen to share my early retreat experience prior to trekking Guatemala here. I believe in leading by example! I think of my time between my trip to the Land of Enchantment, New Mexico, to Mexico, as a mammoth steppingstone. A coming of age filled with mystical, magical moments that have shapeshifted me with a malleable presence inspiring confidence, courage and compassion while sensing a lineage throughout.

In 1979, I first arrived with friend, Jenny B., out of the Midwest suburbs into the desert and mountains of Taos. Our first night was at her friend, Dennis's place. He was an amazing guitar maker whose alluring stone inlays were precious gifts sold to many famous musicians. He offered for us to stay in a gypsy wagon—which was exactly that! I recall writing in my journal the "Scorpio rising, it isn't surprising" poem, which invoked the unusual circumstances and present anticipation of the unknown I was experiencing. In the morning, we opened the wooden doors and *wow*! The clear, dynamic view of the Sacred Mountain of the Pueblo Indians. A sacred memory.

We helped to mud walls of the adobe house projects, made sage bundles, and visited the Puebloans; my favorite being the artists who work and display their beautiful jewelry on the government plaza in Santa Fe. The churches were a cooling, serene sanctuary from the intense afternoon heat and enveloped my prayers in a familiar way.

This was my initiation upon this sacred land, which felt like a protective father energy. The Sacred Mountain of the Pueblo Indians felt as a guardian and gave me strength to endure and continue my journey. This land I would return to often and in the 1980s, being influenced by Susan Harper and her outdoor adventure retreats, I, too, would begin to lead others to this remarkable powerful vortex.

The days ahead involved meeting new friends in a Native American sweat lodge and my first radio interview with a local station. My first of countless radio interviews I have enjoyed throughout my vocation around the country and locally in my hometown Cincinnati. Hiking the desert landscapes in the sweltering afternoon sun, seeing the Milky Way and billions of stars on a typical Taos eve, visits to Ojo Caliente hot springs to renew the body, mind, heart, spirit were among the ways a Taos resident often spent their days. Meeting at Michael's Kitchen, or The Plum Tree Café to hear the music of Eliza Gilkinson, and floating on an innertube from the Rio Grande Bridge down the river to Pilar was another adventure of great courage and maybe stupidity. *I realize I'm lucky to be here typing about it now!*

Women Will Retreat

I taught meditation classes in addition to many hatha yoga classes in the 1980s. When one completed Meditation I & II sessions at the Discovery Center in Cincinnati, they would then be invited to my home where we continued deeper explorations with somatic movement, sound, meditations. From this continued group experience, the spark of an adventure began.

While sponsoring Continuum Movement retreats in Cincinnati led by Susan Harper, we co-taught one near Serpent Mound, an Ohio native earthwork. All these retreats were overnights and created a community of movers and shakers of consciousness. I also taught my own weekend retreats with yoga and somatic movement and breathwork/play of different lengths. More people were becoming involved, and the retreats were inviting a deeper dive into oneself with a sense of exploring self and community and purpose. With "open attention" seeking a new evolutionary and perhaps revolutionary way of yoga and somatic blends into a vital inner dance of life and spirit!

People are the jewels of remembrance and reflection, but you should always extract what you can from a place you're learning and growing in too.

All retreats were held in various buildings in Greater Cincinnati area and always with beautiful surroundings to explore and include in some of the inner work. Still, I longed for the type of adventure Susan experienced with groups out in the wilderness. My dream-time has always been a source of teaching and showing me my next door opening. This was no exception.

Enchantment called! I announced to all my meditation and yoga groups that I would be leading a five-day retreat in Chaco Canyon, New Mexico. I asked that they think and day/night dream about it being a possibility for them too. This was the extent of my marketing. And so, the first Chaco Canyon adventure was created with ten participants in our first group.

We met to list all needs to pack, as this was truly an outdoor adventure with tent camping at Chaco Canyon for a few days. We were all sharing our dreams regarding this and began our journals long before the trip commenced.

I arrived in New Mexico for a few days before to get acclimated, visit friends and prepare to pick up the participants, who arrived from across the country, in the rented fifteen-passenger van at the Albuquerque Airport. Everything revolved around group; this is why solo trekking in Guatemala as part of my evolution was so ecstatic, so surreal. It wasn't simply being in exotica.

I recall listening to their introductions with each other in the van and wondering what our conversations returning would be like. After lunch, we went to the Whole Foods and selected what we might like for our few days in the Chaco Canyon to eat and this was quite the decision-making fiasco. It would be the first and last time I did it in this manner! We gathered our supplies in coolers in the back of the van and headed to Bernalillo, New Mexico to spend our first night in cabins at the KOA. This was a gentle way to slip into the outdoor experience.

The memories from the Southwest retreats elicit deep-belly laughter, recalling pancake breakfast outdoors, a parrot who sat on my shoulder, and our evening fireside gatherings with the Motherpeace Tarot deck. We selected intuitively from the deck a card each day to keep that day on our journey, to dream with at night and awaken with silence each morning gathering in our dream circle sharing. This was a new experience for most, but I have to say, every single person was so ripe and ready to dive into the wild with me.

Morning gatherings summoned the sacred witness within each of us, honoring our sister on her sacred journey. The array of ages, backgrounds, retired and working in so many diverse fields, parents, grandparents, no children, single, etc. brewed quite an eclectic sharing of wisdom.

We drove up to Chaco Canyon onto the bumpy, dirt road to enter, and paused. I placed an audio tape of Clarissa Pinkola Estes reciting from her epic book, *Women Who Run with the Wolves*. We listened to her enchanting tales of women reclaiming their powerful birthright of intuition and wildness. Their innate wisdom and power that so often is repressed in a patriarchal society and imposed even more with patriarchal religious beliefs, rules, and regulations.

As we bumped along the deep ruts on the road, we were aware of the hairpin turn into the canyon and approaching Fajade Butte in Chaco Culture National Historical Park. The hairpin turn with a fifteen-passenger van is always a gulping moment. The silence and listening to Clarissa's tales set a tone for deeper listening and feeling.

With the ranger station in sight, we got out and stretched, babbling about our activities in the canyon of the ancient Anasazi over the next few days.

Once we set up our camp site, helping each other with tents, we all felt called to explore the kiva as a ritual birthing into our new selves, chanting, singing, laughing, and crying. Yoga and meditation started at 6:30 a.m. We hiked to find our spot for our individual practice. Each woman, high atop a mesa overlooking hundreds of miles of vista of the ancient Anasazi, practiced the breathing and spinal moves with an inspiring spaciousness one experiences when practicing in the wide-open spaces of earth.

We returned to our 7:30 silent sharing session with our Motherpeace Tarot card and journal. Breakfast was so delicious outdoors, and everyone took turns creating and cleaning up. Our community evolved while in prayer, in chores, and camaraderie.

Each day, we trekked a different hike and site of the Anasazi roadways, kivas and canyon for five or six hours. Pueblo Bonito with the aligned doorways was a spectacular site. The cylindrical formations seemed to invite the female energy of our group to enter and perform ritual. This was before they closed some of the kivas due to preservation. We hiked the high mesas and petro-glyph trails to the Super Nova, shaman-stained petroglyph high above the mesa where the winds would nearly blow us off the wall.

When standing atop the canyon, the vista of hundreds of miles totally opens your body-mind-heart with a spaciousness not experienced in the confines of rooms or cities. That is why taking your body out into the wilderness and allowing the beauty and wildness of nature to tap into you is an extraordinary, lifetime spiritual high. Not getting high but a sustaining being high.

We had fun taking artistic photos of yoga poses on cliffs within the doorway frames of a stone kiva. We were rained upon walking on slippery pathways and sun-kissed on warm sandy stones as a tribe experiencing the ancient landscapes of women before us. Sometimes it felt so familiar. The touch, the scent of the sage, the dry desert sun and oh, the Milky Way heavenly sky landscapes on the cold evenings. We were sketching, water coloring, photographing, journaling and just absorbing, soaking it all in as best we could. The open-air wildness of exploring an ancient culture initiated our tribe into spiraling vortex of energies, the intensity of the weather, the altitude, the land, the cultural history and spirit here in Chaco Canyon infused our chakras with a spinning electrical current and creating new ways of seeing, engaging and knowing. Wisdom of the ages streamed through our energetic veins, and our hearts and minds and bodies were excited!

After dinner, we would head out to a particular kiva for a silent sunset meditation. The celestial light show was our visual dessert moments. These were such a sacred delight, visually with the dramatic sunsets, and internally as a moment of connection with the universe. Our psyches now so wide open to take in the magnificence and wonders of the earth's rotation from day to nightfall. The sounds of nightfall, crows cawing an eerie sensation echoing of canyon walls, coyote howls and whatever you may imagine hearing scurrying near your tent sometimes kept you awake.

After a few days, we headed out to Ojo Caliente, stopping for lunch at a roadside stand in Abiquiu, New Mexico near Georgia

O'Keefe's homebase in the southwest. As I write this, I picture each of the three groups I experienced over the years, sitting at this same picnic table sharing food, stories and abundant laughter.

Mud baths were my special gooey luxury at Ojo, a massage and soaking in the various pools. We stayed here overnight and hiked up behind the springs into the hills. We then went off onto our own with journals, watercolors and meditating in silence with the scent of sage, sandstone and clay pottery chards here and there along the pathway. Ojo holds a special place in my heart.

Our drive through the green landscape was a healing sight from the stark sun within the canyon walls at Chaco. The flowers in bloom greeted us with many colors. I purposely took these trips during September for the flowering beauty in the mountains and the weather.

Over the Rio Grande bridge, turn left at the then yellow blinking light to Jenny B.'s winding dirt road, another feat for the van to her lovely home and beautiful sage landscape. Our retreat always involved a meditation, prayer and ritual beneath the earth in her underground kiva. This was another pivotal moment for all on these southwest journeys. We sat on the mudded seating, drumming, chanting, singing, passing the prayer stick around to invite a vocal input to Spirit. We danced on the dirt floor, created silent moments to feel into and when ready as a group experience, we climbed the wooden kiva ladder, and opened the earthen doorway lid to the light of day. A birthing out into the world, seeing the Sacred Mountain in the distance at the Pueblo was a blessing from this sacred land.

If time and the Pueblo permitted, we would visit the oldest living and functioning pueblo in our world, the Taos Pueblo. The aroma of bread baking in the clay ovens, the stunning jewelry of turquoise and coral and silver, and ceremonial dances were an amazing highlight of our journey. We always ended this part of the journey with breakfast at Michael's Kitchen, then off to Santa Fe for a few hours.

We returned to the KOA for our last evening together. Our new tribe held ceremony and chose our last Motherpeace card for our last morning dreamtime gathering. Sharing of dreams was absolutely mind-blowing with images that prompted us to create healthy, lasting changes in our lives, honor all of who we are on this earth this lifetime and go in peace, with courage and enthusiasm back into our daily walk.

The drive in the van to the airport was a lot different than the arrival. Our stories were of heroic feats and heartfelt courage to explore what we thought we could not. A tribe was created. Each group I had the blessing and privilege to share this remarkable spiritual landscape and possibilities with inspired new avenues for growth and sisterhood.

REACH AND RECEIVE: REFLECTION

Pause to reflect on an insurmountable goal you achieved. On paper or in your mind, list what it took to accomplish it and how it contributed to your growth. Note how you feel as you stop to give yourself recognition. This recognition acts in your being as cumulative self-love, resilience, and courage.

Chapter 11

Giant Leap into Best Self

"Life shrinks or expands according to one's courage."

—ANAIS NIN

JUMPING OFF THE cliff into unknown territory often is not how I would characterize myself, but now, you have drastic examples of me doing this. Perhaps most spontaneous was leaping into the sky with parachuting! My friend, Jenny B. and I took a deep breath and sighed into this new adventure of parachuting one autumn in the outskirts of Cincinnati. I would be turning thirty in a few weeks and parachuting just seemed to be the perfect way to initiate a new decade. With not just one but two emergency landings. I highly recommend it as way to explore the earth through jumping out of a plane, total surrender to your jump master/guide and your parachute, and float in awe of Mother Earth's beauty.

With just a few hours of practice at the nearby parachuting center, one is prepared and ready to slip into the suit, buckle up the chute on your back and the reserve chute on your chest. This

117

was the only training! Trusting in your jumpmaster who you just met is essential as well.

I boarded the small prop plane with my instructor and the pilot who already had the place warmed up. I sat beside the pilot and the opened window near the wing as we flew up to about 3,400 feet. My instructor was drilling me with questions, which I nervously would answer when the pilot mentioned to him, I had my arm wrapped around the pilot's leg! Not sure what I was thinking, but I was clearly resisting turning toward to opened window and jumping out of this plane.

Door, pedal, jump was the command in a quick one, two, three and leap into the air! I did to my amazement and floated with ease. It was autumn. The colors of the trees below reminded me of a bowl of Fruit Loops. I had a radio attached and was supposed to receive instructions on which toggle to pull so I would land at the airport. I was in awe of the sensation of floating and seeing. The whisper of the wind was so calming and the beauty of the earth stunning. Suddenly I realized I was floating over a subdivision, noticed an inground pool, utility wires above the county road, a barn and oh dear, a bull in the yard!

My parachuting suit was a bright red and white checkered covering, which I'm sure the bull thought was quite a gift floating toward him. Now, in yoga, one is taught to repeat your mantra when you are aware of pending death. It was a fifty-fifty chance of which toggle to yank on to lift myself over the top of the barn and landing couple feet from barbed wire fencing. When I landed near a little lady's backyard during my first jump, I certainly wasn't exclaiming out loud my mantra upon my landing! The lady was doing dishes and heard my screaming expletive, looked out her window and saw me floating into her yard. She was the first to greet me.

The people at the airport watched as I floated away, got in their cars and rushed to the retrieval scene. Apparently, my radio was not working! But hey, I survived. Would I ever do this again? That leap off the plane pedal was one of the most surrendering energies I have ever experienced. I went home and breathed a lot that week in November, reliving the moment of the bull, utility wires and the emergency landing. Would I ever be able to parachute again? Yes! I got right back up the following Saturday in the prop plane, nervously turning toward the open window, foot on pedal and leapt out into the open sky again! This time landing in a soybean gushy. muddy field for a soft landing but away from the airport again. My jumpmaster was ill that day, so I had another guy who happened to spot me wrongly. I noticed but this time, saw the open field and was able to direct the parachute for a landing in a farmer's field.

I highly recommend the experience as it is certainly a test of courage, surrender and navigation. However, I will never venture again into the skies for a giant leap out of a plane!

REACH AND RECEIVE: STRETCH

Do you need to leap today? If you have been putting off "parachuting" into a challenge, believe you have the skills to move through it. The outcome might surprise you. Facing our fears or even doing a different activity stretches us into newfound knowledge, emotions and stories to share. The activity may even replace a bad habit or limiting belief.

Chapter 12

Foundations and Forums for Healing

"It is only with the heart that one can see rightly; what is essential is invisible to the eye."

—ANTOINE DE SAINT-EXUPERY

POSSESS YEARS OF intense study from world-renowned teachers of yoga, meditation and somatic movement at this point. And I want to impress, as a teacher, I feel it is of paramount importance to explain my methods and philosophy and pass them on. I practice what I teach with regards to a daily effort in continuing to learn through exploring in my own practice/sadhana. I continue to learn from my peers and when I do share what I learned, I always give credit to the teachers who shared with me. When I discover from my own practice and share with my students/teacher trainees, I also tell them it was from my entering a practice with the openness of an adventurous explorer.

A concern I have these past few years is regarding yoga teacher training programs. Some are conducted with persons being *certified* with a 200-hour program and then sharing as an expert, even giving teacher trainings. Also, yoga teacher training becoming a major business venture to bring needed support revenue to sustain a yoga studio. Sharing with others to become a yoga teacher is a lifetime mentorship and vocation for me. And I could not even have imagined inviting this sharing for many years, decades perhaps. Even then, I would consult with my teachers and acknowledge their counsel while engaging in sharing this ancient wisdom with another. When I have been approached to teach someone, help guide them for a lifetime of yoga teaching, I search within myself if my heart is resonating with their heart on this matter. I search to hear of a vocation call rather than a career. I have shared with integrity and grace, mentoring those who have such a calling and will continue always with enthusiasm and a devotion when called upon.

My dear friends reading this, know being a yoga teacher is a great responsibility. Physically, mentally, emotionally, spiritually you are inviting an openness into one's deep self. This needs to be met with someone experienced because of their own in-depth inner work—and one who practices with a daily sadhana that deepens their connection in myriad ways.

For example, physically, I enter my practice noticing my left shoulder is tight and explore with yoga moves and somatic movement and breaths to enter this tightness and feel the shift to lighten this tightness. This may sound mundane, but this inquiry offers you enormous opportunity to seek and feel the change you can create. Sharing this with my students during a session encourages their exploration and gives them hope to be their own teacher of their unique practice each day. It empowers them to do so and trust their own intuition!

For another example, mentally, I enter my practice feeling so scattered in my thoughts, depressed, emotionally drained from some instance. I initiate my practice to clear the clutter of thought with breath and meditation and always incorporating movement. I feel more in my body than out of body with constant chatter in my mind, which is an escape from embodiment. Embodiment is being aligned, whole, and balanced. I can share with students who suffer from depression or just having a bad day overall, the way yoga and movement meditation can aid in lightening the density. It encourages them to explore in this way. Imbedded traumas can shift and lighten the density, lighten trauma's hold, free the body-mind-heart to breathe spaciously again, and feel happiness enter through the tributaries of our organic malleable body. Strength and resilience surface with confidence and balance.

Finally, spiritually, I might feel so removed, scattered and disconnected from a sacred source in my life. So, in my practice, perhaps with the daily Sacred Heart sequence, I realign and remember my breath as an umbilical cord to a sacred source.

A deep connection with bountiful blessings is made possible by a simple practice. And, so my dear friend, who may be a teacher/student, know the immense value and opportunity for learning lies directly with your engagement with YOU! Each day, you are the source of teaching, wisdom, esoteric knowledge of being human on this spinning planet. You will be of valuable resource to your students when properly mentored by another who has walked this path and deeply explored, and most importantly, through your devotion to your daily, yes daily, vocational practice of yoga! The source of your inspiration lies within YOU!

A valued teacher knows daily sadhana is the way.

Forums for Healing

There are many ways I have expressed myself as teacher and pioneered new avenues for new possibilities for yoga, somatic movement, and meditation to be shared and valued. Here is a sequence from my early days to present day. You cannot know how this excites me to see and witness! I also share here for you to be inspired to create your own legacy. Remember, the seed of mine started in my living room fifty years ago, in front of a television, stretching next to a cat.

Substitute Teaching: An Initiation for New Teachers

My first experience was substitute teaching for Lilias in her classes at the high school for an adult education program. The articulation was seemingly flawless and spewed with ease from my psyche out into the vast auditorium filled to brim with yoga mats and participants upon them. I was amazed at how this felt so comfortable and familiar!

I was in my element so to speak, nervously excited, but upon the first few sentences of instruction felt enormous support from my teacher, Lilias.

Substitute teaching is a great way to notice *what you do not know* too! You may find a need for notes, a need to outline to feel secure and find the questions from participants you cannot answer confidently all are prompts to learn more from your teachers, study and from within yourself, your practice. To teach with confidence is to be a student for life! Do you have that commitment?

Family Health Program (FHP)

This idea came to me in a dream as often the inspirations do. Often, one person from a family unit is studying, practicing and gaining benefits from their practice in body-mind-heart-spirit. After a session, one returns home more so to a partner, family unit. Yes, of course, singles practice too! My point is when we return there is a "reentry" process most times where one needs to be alone be it for a few minutes or hours. This new program idea seemed to help with the isolation of being the only one within a family practicing and benefiting and would create a healthier family unit in many ways.

My inspired nudging was about creating a way for a whole family engagement in a simple yet deeply effective practice. Children are easily able to absorb the energy of a practice having less layered tensions, anxieties, and preconceptions. This idea was relentless in its composition in my mind and enthusiasm! I invited a few well- respected, trusted friends in the holistic work to listen and give feedback with this idea. "Nothing like it" I would hear repeatedly with encouragement to continue in its creation.

I recall creating logos and descriptions. In a dream, I saw the logo with the letters "FHP" staggered below each other and connected. With a black magic marker, I drew the image and typed the description on typing paper with a Royal typewriter! Pleased with its appearance, off I went to the Milford Print Shop and had it copied onto light yellow paper for distribution around town.

That was the "marketing" back in the day. No online presence, webinars, Zoom and Facebook ads with professional graphic designers. Just carry your box of flyers from the printer to various storefronts to post on bulletin boards, talk about with staff so they can spread the word, and find posting on poles in university area neighborhoods to staple flyers. Also, I would include direct mail to other yoga teachers, holistic health presenters and holistic medical personnel with a personal letter to get the word out. This was the way I advertised my work throughout the 70s and into mid-80s. With this FHP program, I also sent the program info and availability out to therapists in the field of psychology.

One family participating was a single mother with a couple of children. One of her sons was experiencing anger issues and having problems at school. She inquired if I would be willing to work with her and the children. They had spent many hours in psychotherapy together and singularly.

I agreed and wanted her to be sure with him first that he would welcome learning to relax. He said yes with an enthusiasm, to her surprise! Before we met, I focused on him in my practice with healing meditations, surrounding him in lightness of love and its healing potential.

The boy, Robert, arrived, looking a bit scared yet willing. We spent first moments getting to know each other and talked about the wonderful experience of *being calm*. He was curious to have such an experience. We practiced breathing techniques with a simplicity he could use in a practical way throughout his day. We practiced pausing/witnessing our emotions before acting out and using a new tool of breath play, which I shared was a great yogi's special secret. He was curious again and willing and liked the idea of knowing a special yogi's secret. *Shhhhh!* We moved in the curious animal poses of a cat, dog, cobra, lion sigh, a tree for rooting and balance. He enjoyed the playfulness with which we explored these poses in yoga. I met with the family also in our relaxation guiding through layers of tensions, anxieties we were able to experience letting go in yoga sessions that were playful like expressing the lion growl and slithering cobra, balancing like a tree and many other expressions with lightness. We could feel the healing of being calm and playfully light together! It was revolutionary and joyful moment for all, including me.

Because of a dream and following up on it, this family was able to be helped in a deep, meaningful way. They left with lifelong tools to practice being calm, managing stressors and anxieties and being light and playful again.

Drug & Alcohol Rehab Residential Program

I received an invitation to teach yoga within a hospital environment, a residential twenty-eight-day drug/alcohol rehab program. This is early 1980s and to share yoga as a possible valuable tool with this group was both a challenge and an opportunity I was excited to accept.

Once a week, in the evening, I arrived at a local hospital and entered a smoke- filled, jam-packed room of mostly men who were in treatment. We had limited space but as I've always managed to do, I created a formation of participants allowing for a simple routine that required limited spatial necessity. I recall having to sit upon the edge of a table as there was no room for me on the crowded room floor. It all worked out though.

After the first week, I typed up a sheet on my manual typewriter, as the participants wanted a handout of the yoga routine to follow when I was not there. I drew stick figures to accompany the written instruction. Some used it to practice together with throughout the week.

The relaxation was said to be the most calming and healing moment for many. It was reassuring they could use yoga breathing, pranayama, to assist in their daily recovery. Along with simple six spinal flow movements, lying down, sitting, standing, it was a simple yet very effective in creating internal balance.

I truly feel the response was so well-received by participants because they FELT better! I would point out that "getting high and being high" are two very different vibrations of our human potential.

Yoga is all about "being in a high vibration frequency" and it is our birthright. They received glimpses of this somatic felt vibration and would express how their bodies felt light and not so burdened physically and mentally. They shared how their anxious moments were able to be addressed with new tools and confidence.

Yoga practice, with simple spinal asanas, deep spacious breathing and a very soothing relaxation can be a valuable healing modality in one's recovery. Yoga creates a balance in our chemistry relating to our endocrine immune systems. If you practice a few moments each day, you will visibly see and internally feel positive changes in your body and your mind and deeply within your heart.

Yoga in a Gym

Oh, the feedback I received when asked to teach at a Gold's Gym! I was told I could not teach yoga in such an environment, as it would not be respected and would have to be a watered-down version. If I agreed, I could not possibly be true to yoga principles! This is an exact phrase from another teacher to me.

I was in my forties and met a personal physical trainer one day. We had a delightful sharing of our expertise and wanted to experience each other's way of caring for the body. So, Michael trained me on weights, machines, floor work and I shared yoga with him. He was amazed at core strength possibilities with yoga, and I was amazed at the addition of using weights, etc. to enhance my strength and good health.

While on various machines, I would also share with him ways someone's posture could be helpful or detrimental to what they may want to achieve. For example, I noticed so many with improper sitting, tailbones/shoulder blades away from seat and back of machine would strain eventually various spinal areas. Also, while standing and lifting hand weights I pointed out how so many would extend and use their neck in the lifts.

We both enjoyed learning and exchanging. And look at today! Yoga is taught at every gym anywhere, everywhere! I also began working with other trainers and their clients personally. I would witness their routine and give them needed alignment cues, particular asanas relating to help with certain tight areas, or injury recovery. I continue this work today and find it immensely satisfying.

Introducing yoga to various corporate entities like P&G, financial institutions, health facilities, attorney offices, brokerage firms, special corporate group meetings and their gyms has continued. I have never compromised in my yoga sharing to "fit in" a gym setting. As a matter of fact, I enjoy creating safe, comfortable, peaceful settings within gym settings. Dimming lights, encircling the group, and always with a sacred heart influencing our practice together. Teaching is such a joy for me no matter the setting.

Yoga and Holistic Health in Corporations and Hospitals

In 1994, I received a phone call from Jeanette, an RN with a hospital medical corporation which had just built and opened a spacious health club facility. She requested my expertise to be with a handful of others in various fields to create a Holistic Health branch for this medical health corporation. She told me my name came up in many meetings and conversations and she was eager to speak with me. We made an appointment to meet and share possibilities in this new creation and after our first meeting, I was so excited to be a part of this great new adventure! The medical doctor, Steve, along with six people representing various aspects from biofeedback, nutrition, healing touch, yoga and meditation, tai chi were all enthused to be a part of this new project for TriHealth Corporation, their clients, patients and staff. The luxurious grand health pavilion was a gorgeous sight to behold too!

At our beginning, we had an off-site house turned into studio with office and open space for movement. I held private and class offerings here for a while until we were offered space within the new health pavilion. On the third floor, away from the hustle and bustle of the ground floor and second floor with trainers, swimmers, all gym facilities and participants, we were quietly nestled in our own space with ambient music, essential oil diffusing for a more holistic environment. We held private sessions and shared the space harmoniously. We had a front desk administrative assistant, Karen, who was so efficient in providing for all our needs for a smooth functioning program. It was rapidly becoming known throughout Cincinnati, Kentucky and Indiana.

One of the many benefits was learning from each other

scientific findings and approaches in holistic modules of health and sharing this valuable research with participants. Marketing was a specialty for corporate health facilities, so we had full access to a wide range of strategies to get the word out.

I conducted numerous radio interviews on a local NPR station over the years for TriHealth and loved participating in radio. I was called often when a guest could not show up! Also, we had TV interviews over the years on various topics. It also nudged us to be well-informed on the latest research and to step up with professionalism and authenticity, which we displayed during and after each occasion to share via media.

We were well established as a professional holistic model for others locally and nationally to emulate, just as CYTA was in the 70s. Our number of participants for individual sessions and classes were growing so we moved my classes to a hospital environment, which had a large area for movement. One class turned into two and more throughout the week.

Also, I was asked if I could create a class for expectant mothers. I consulted with an OB-GYN regarding some of the movements for modifications and regarding any considerations for mother and baby. Thus, the first prenatal yoga class was created! I taught it at the local hospitals for a couple of years. I trained other yoga teachers to use this as a model for future prenatal sessions privately and in classes.

We also had participants who had injuries unable to get on the floor but wanted to try yoga. So, a chair yoga class was created where we would use the chair from sitting to support while standing and modifying with chair support such poses as triangle, tree, warrior, and my very own creation, which I still share today in each class, the "kitchen sink" pose! We were growing quickly and eventually, we were not able to accommodate the number of participants who inquired to sign up. There was a meeting of the holistic group on the third floor with the health facility group on the first floor and we were able to use their expansive room for our yoga classes. Members of the facility could get for free I believe while nonmembers paid. All would have to sign up in advance and be at the door fifteen minutes before class to sign in as we had a cut-off of fifty, yes, fifty people. The line was long when I arrived and unfortunately, some would not get to enter because of fire regulations.

The yoga mats were of a thick Styrofoam type and slipped on the floor. I begged for sticky yoga mats for safety precautions and eventually got them. These classes were one of firsts in health facilities locally and nationally. Yoga was becoming very popular for providing healthful benefits for their members. The way I taught was blending a somatic sense of being and exploring and was very different from other yoga classes offered. My Continuum study and practice in the years before was integrated within my sharings as a unique way, a welcoming way, a devotional way of being in your body and exploring with yoga. Including wave motion, with deep, open attention and a soothing relaxation always at the end of each class, just as Lilias Folan offered decades before.

Soon, I was offered many other corporate opportunities for classes and workshops throughout the city once my pilot Proctor & Gamble holistic model for classes took off within their facilities. They were just beginning to create gym facilities on sites and while under construction, I would hold sessions in small meeting rooms where we were quite crowded but had so much fun too. I also taught at corporations, financial institutions, brokerage firms, lawyers' firms, and other places.

Retreats within these corporations offsite were one of my favorite sharings. Removed from the work environment into a natural setting with the beauty of nature embracing the deeper inner work was a specialty I so enjoy! Where the participants could shed the daily all-consuming workloads, the stances of power structures and all be together in a circle unfolding, unwinding and remembering their passions and purposes beyond their jobs! This is so rewarding in so many ways and layers. Including yoga and holistic modalities in a health program not only enriches this experience in deep, layered movements for healing but can improve quality of work.

While I write of these experiences, I am reminded of people who appeared in my life from other avenues of health-related fields to study and mentor and eventually take a teacher training with me. From Zumba instructors and kickboxing, it was a staff who honored and respected each other. With a kickboxing crew, I created a day workshop of the best of both dynamics blended. We had a blast teaching together. Again, this was a first to offer these two modalities in a blend of large spatial movements with direct intention and the subtle gentle flow and exploration of yoga. All who attended loved it.

Recordings

After classes in the 1980s, many would ask if they could bring a tape recorder to class so they could record and take home. After a while, it was challenging because I would not want to be stationary near a recording device certainly not the quality of today. I sought out a recording studio, created a script and recorded a relaxation tape for students, *Breath of New Life*. I was amazed at its popularity! Other requests for a hatha yoga session were received and I recorded a simple beginner's class. *Align and Awaken* was another recording requested by continuing students. I even had students request specific poses they hoped to be in the class recording. This now was on a CD, and I am still told people are sharing this and using it to practice in their homes. I enjoyed being in the studios and recording. It just always felt natural and relaxing to do so.

Cancer Support Community (formerly The Wellness Community)

This avenue of opportunity is so very special. As of this writing, I am still serving the valuable practice of exploring yoga for this community.

It was 1994 and I received another phone call. The call was from Sherry W., a partner with Lynn Stern in creation of the Cincinnati-based The Wellness Center (TWC), which offered free programs for cancer patients and their support people.

At this time, they were sharing support group processes with social workers and therapists leading the discussions on lung, ovarian, breast, colon, pancreatic cancer. Each would be unique in the information for the participants. It was a valued sacred space so all could share their situations and receive support psychologically as well as a new community of friends.

I was asked to come in and talk with Lynn about adding another element, yoga.

They wanted to include a holistic health module to their offerings. Also, they contacted a known Tai Chi teacher.

We discussed the difference in the language of "healing" and "curing", and I was very specific about being clear with all participants how this could be a valuable tool for so many layers in their journey. My beginnings with this group were experiencing a caring, supportive and knowledgeable staff who had a great sense of humor and just a delight to be with. Almost thirty years later, this remains so true! A different staff now but the continued resonance of joyful comradery and support. This is a space for healing for all, even the staff who work here.

As we began introducing yoga classes to the schedule along with Tai Chi, the Wellness Center was becoming a popular center practicing holistic health in Cincinnati area for cancer patients, family members and support persons. Also, the staff would participate! This was so helpful in a couple of ways. One, they were receiving the benefits of yoga personally and, secondly, could through their first-hand experience pass on information to others they came in contact with about their personal benefits as well as hearing comments from participants on how they felt afterward and during the week because of yoga. We even had board members showing up in class from time to time.

At this point of TWC offerings, they were residing in a donated space of a bank building, with an entire floor available. It was furnished functionally with the yoga and Tai Chi sessions held in an open, carpeted space with lovely windows allowing light to filter in. At some point, we were then downsized in space and my yoga classes were in a furnished small living room area. We made it work though! A few of the participants would enjoy lying on the sofas for deep relaxation practice. We would use the chairs in ways of support for those in treatment who were feeling side effects such as nausea, swelling and other discomfort. But they would keep showing up because they felt much better afterward!

Somewhere down the road, Lynn, the director had a vision and had sponsors to make her vision of a beautiful free-standing building with abundant rooms for support sessions, spacious kitchen and area for yoga and Tai Chi, a library providing a variety of supportive information for crucial health decisions, for inspiration and raising one's spirit during this intense moment in their life. A spacious parking lot and a lovely porch for continued relaxations and conversations that developed into very supportive meaningful relationships. To this day, participants enjoy sitting and talking with each other after a class or session. The Adirondack rockers are especially enjoyable for after session tea and conversations. Lynn realized her vision!

I recall in the later 90s when preparing for a TV segment interview for TWC, I came across a psych article from NIH regarding a new avenue of psychoneuroimmunology. Well, that was a mouthful for body, mind, immune connection study. So, I used this term during my interview commenting about how medical science is confirming what yogis of ancient times knew—how yoga and its engagement with wholeness of a person, how yoga moves (asanas), correlate with endocrine glands, immune health, and the value of deep relaxation, along with deep, spacious oxygenating breaths are of paramount importance in bringing one to balance.

Once I begin sharing in interviews or talks to groups such as Breast Cancer Alliance, I am on a roll with a passionate fervor to bridge the ancient teachings with present-day science in my presentations! I just so enjoy sharing the value of this amazing vast healthful system of yoga!

So many participants throughout these thirty years I have served here, have breathed and moved and relaxed with me. In the early days of TWC and my entry into the world of sharing with persons some who were terminally ill, some were support angels, I was treading upon a path so new yet very rewarding. The delicate nature of being neutral with empathy and compassion is quite a soulful practice. It became such a retreat for many, and the class participant numbers continued to increase.

Each class was an exploration of learning what aspects of yoga and breaths were helpful for the individuals and their treatments for a variety of cancer diagnoses. I learned about ports and other tubing, chemo and radiation side effects, blood pressure changes, deep aching, nausea and numbness. What poses may be contradictive in providing comfort and movements with breaths that would provide energy and a nurturing calming. There was no precedence for this thus far, and it was an invaluable experience for us all to learn together! What courage the first participants and present-day participants have when walking in for a session. So many are coming to their first ever yoga class!

Over these many years, I have developed a curriculum not in a standard one-size-fits-all format, but first, a way of seeing and listening that guides the teacher and students to accommodate for a beneficial experience. In a class, you will have participants with brain cancer, breast cancer, prostate cancer, colon cancer with colostomy bags and so on. What props are comfortable and which ones are not is very important information.

Lynn, the director, was such a caring mentor for me. Her heartfelt guidance and expertise from both being a director and a cancer patient herself was a rich field to learn and grow in. One afternoon, when I entered the building for our yoga session the receptionist said she wanted to see me in her office before I started class. I entered and immediately felt her spacious heart through her eyes. She stood up from behind her desk to give me a hug and to share that one of my enthusiastic participants, Ann, a triathlete, young mother of a three-year-old, had passed on during the weekend. In Lynn's office was a poster of Ann with her dynamic laughter and strong presence. I told her with tears, Ann had called me before I left to teach a weekend yoga retreat and she shared how much I and our session meant to her. She didn't want to tell me she was in hospice and nearing her passing because she knew it would affect my retreat. Her friend and support person shared this with me later.

The personal heart-inspiring and heart-breaking stories over thirty years have enriched me in ways I could not have imagined when I began. I am truly blessed to be of service with this community.

So many have shared deep stories of their courage, fears, happiness and sadness, family and friend stories over the years. I have laughed deep belly laughter and cried with so many. I have attended many celebrations; some that were their memorials. So many hearts opened mine and I tear up now remembering quite a few of these special angels who, since 1994 to present-day, gifted me with their presence. I have experienced other participants or their families calling me to let me know how much our yoga practice was a gift for them. How the breath and relaxation is so helpful for them at the end of their life to relax and let go. I have had families give me special treasures which my students wanted them to give me after their passing. I have all of these gifts on an altar and value remembering their light, their heart, their courage and resilience.

I was asked years ago by a former staff person who I ran into at a coffee shop, how can I continue after all these years, don't I get depressed? All I know is this service is very dear to my heart, partly because of Lynn Stern who herself passed on and I attended her memorial; partly because of these participant—some who arrive being terminally ill looking for peace and comfort, others who bring family/friends for support; and valuing the term "survivor" and living it as vibrantly as possible. Another very meaningful reason is my own mother, Dorothy, and her diagnosis and journey in her forties with cancer. The was back in the sixties and there was no support system organization until a year or so later. Her amazing strength and resilience and loving kindness as she offered herself for research for chemo and radiation (which back then was radium insertions. I dedicate this service to her and dedicated my book to her also.

Cancer Support Community is a healing place where those affected by cancer either as a patient or support person can gather to take their mind off the stress of being recently diagnosed or in treatment. All who come and continue to lie on their yoga mats each week glean some benefit, inspire me each class, each week, each month and year and decade!

Each week, when I enter the building and begin setting up the room with mats, I am eager to see who will enter through the doors. This is a safe space for all, those who choose various treatments, those who choose no treatment, the support persons, some who are grieving, some who feel vulnerable and some who feel a warrior spirit. All are welcomed in a circle of caring support and compassion.

Lynn Stern is most definitely smiling at her creation and vision and mostly because she knew the value it would bring to so many. Thousands and thousands have benefitted from the *free* programs these many years and it is exciting to see it continue to unfold and grow. The portrait of Lynn that her husband, Ned, painted hangs in the living room of this beautiful facility. It makes me smile to see her. I was mentored by the best. I now must wipe my tears and pause. With love I pause. With amazing facial memories of many who entered my classes over the decades, their stories of hopes and fears, their courage and warriorlike attitude with diagnosis, these people are teachers who continue to grace my life.

Select Presentations and Programs

Chanting Mantra Sound

Indian Cultural Festival, University of Cincinnati

Cincinnati Health Expo, Cincinnati, Fountain Square Plaza

Day of Yoga, Annual Event/Fundraiser, CYTA

Midwest Music Therapy Association, Cincinnati, Ohio

Sensory Expansion Workshops, Co-taught with Kathy Hunter, Cincinnati, Ohio

Mantra and Sounding Healing, Private and Group Sessions

Tuning Fork Solfeggio Frequencies Vibrational Healing, Private and Group Sessions

Yoga Somatic Movement Meditation

Inner Dance, Discovery Center, Cincinnati, Ohio

Body Play, Discovery Center, Cincinnati, Ohio

Meditation 1 & 2, Discovery Center, Cincinnati, Ohio

Inner Dance of Yoga, Classes for Contemporary Dance Theatre, Cincinnati, Ohio

Women and Anger Workshops, Co-taught with Aja Linda Griffin, MS, LC, Beavercreek, Ohio

Women and Anger Workshop, Co-taught with Dr. Susan Crew, Ph.D., Cincinnati, Ohio

Love's Body Emerges Workshops, Co-taught with Kate Jones, Cincinnati and San Francisco, California

Love's Body Emerges Workshops, Co-Taught with Vickie Fairchild, PT, Cincinnati, Ohio

Calming Presence of Yoga, Ongoing Classes and Workshops

Lectures

St. Joseph Infant Home Womens Guild

Mt. St. Joseph College, Cincinnati, Womens Studies Program

Mt. Notre Dame High School, Career Day Main Presenter

Northern Kentucky University

Pacifica University, San Francisco (slide presentation, Guatemala journey)

Proctor & Gamble, Speaker, Holistic Health/Relaxation/ Meditation and Women Executive Offsite

Retreats

Spiritual Frontier Fellowship National, Coco Beach, Florida

Villa Serena, Co-taught with Lilias, Sarasota, Florida

Immaculate Heart of Mary Center, Continuum Movement, Yoga, Meditation, Monroe, Michigan

Power of Breath, Co-taught with Kamalu, Cincinnati, Ohio

Chapter 13

Summary of a Journey from Chaos to Calm

"Peace comes from within. Do not seek it without."

—BUDDHA

I AM HUMBLED YOU have read my story of a fifty-year journey in yoga and somatic health studies and curious observations of life through the lens of a yogi. I am in awe of the amazing adventures I have had the privilege to partake in. I also am in awe of the wonderful inspiring teachers and mentors I have been blessed with along the way. The valuable friendships with so many others walking their unique path and sharing with me are precious gems in my unfolding.

I reflect on how easy it is nowadays for you to obtain valuable information on yoga and somatic movement for health, and when I was beginning my search, we had to look far and wide for books and information without computers and without the ability to search the Internet and be globally connected within a second.

We could not even have imagined such a possibility back in 1973 when I began my first yoga class. Thus, I have countless books from India's finest teachers of eons ago, from scientist and spiritual mentors. I joke that my kids will be having a holistic yard sale when I exit someday abundant with books and crystals, tuning forks, drums and all items new age. There will be some valuable energized items to be sure.

With the ease and availability with which you can attain knowledge of your body and its miraculous movements and possibilities to live a healthy, vibrant life, is there an excuse that prohibits your *reaching and receiving*?

What will your fifty-year journey be to share? What has inspired you to be a living, vibrant, healthy sacred being on earth this lifetime? What do you want to contribute to the sacred sphere of knowing and being? What is your unique story to be told? I am looking forward to hearing of your wondrous moments of seeing, exploring, creating and connecting.

In Part 2 of this book, the manual, I purposely emphasize the focus of simplicity. It is a basic path for you to immediately initiate a yoga and somatic practice with the deep sacred intention of being all you can be as your Sacred Source intended. Be the miracle you are! The movements and suggestions for breathing are all simple ways to practice, bringing a healthy vibe within your heart-mind-body, and unfold into each day reaching for the abundant energy and receiving the gifts of a brand-new day, for a brand new, awakening moment!

Practice!

Awaken each day feeling the breath and be inspired with each con-scious inhalation and enthused to unfold into your new day with each conscious exhalation. *Reach and Receive* this gift of a new day each and every morning and practice a few moments the pre-cious Sacred Heart Sequence beside your bed. Honor your being in your miraculous body on this miraculous spinning-in-outer-space planet earth this very day. Care with love and compassion for all and who you are.

Again, thank you for reading my story and I hope it may in some way inspire your adventurous journey.

PART II

PRACTICE GUIDE:
PRANA AND POSES

Introduction

Science of Yoga

WHEN I BEGAN my journey into yoga, I was introduced to a plethora of books from India, where, of
course, yoga began. These texts were for extensive training and study at the Yoga Seminary of the spiritual science and the
rich history of this lineage I was becoming involved with. These
books included ancient texts with then modern-day (mid-1900s)
physicians' findings and conclusions based on their research. By
the way, the prices for these books ranged from $1-$3. Imagine
that!

The Science of Pranayama, by Swami Sivananda is one such text
that covered Prana in detail. This book is a layered study of Prana,
sub-Prana, the variation of energy as colors and sounds and mudra
hand positions, the properties for various organs, glands, and auric
fields, and the detailed purification process.

Swamiji Sivananda founded the Divine Life Society in 1936
and among its many facets was the connection with an allo-
pathic hospital offering free medical aid to those suffering and an
Ayurvedic Pharmaceutical Works, which prepares high-quality

ayurvedic medicines that are well-respected around the world. Another facet of health service was an eye hospital that offered and provided treatments at an in-patient facility including free food and medicines. A humbling service created by a yogi doctor to enrich lives with the basic principles of a yoga lifestyle. This includes sharing with unconditional love your fellow inhabitants on earth by the service of dissemination of yoga health…body-mind-heart-spirit. This work is the sacred science that continues to be a creative, caring and constant community for all to receive valuable health benefits.

In the *Science of Pranayama*, Swamiji speaks of letter writing, wireless cables, and traveling on trains and airplanes to distant lands. And to distant lands he sent forth a student, Swami Vivekananda, who would be a main speaker at the World Religion Summit held in Chicago. He became well-known and his writings within his book, *The Complete Works of Yoga*, is an all-encompassing and deep understanding of the many facets of yoga.

Another text that many of us in yoga teacher training in the 1970s acquired for scientific study was *The Complete Book of Yoga*, by Swami Vishnudevananda, a student and disciple of Swamiji Sivananda. This was written in the 1950s and first published in 1960. It is a most comprehensive illustration of science and spirituality of yoga and a great resource for us back in the day. My copy is well-worn but is nonetheless, a continued valuable resource.

I was fascinated by the correlation of the endocrine system with energy centers, chakras. The effects of fields of energy we exist within/without, the simple practices of cleansing, which is vital to our health, and the asanas, the pranayama, Patanjali's *8 Steps of Attaining Yoga (Union)*. I continue to share from this well of knowledge, connecting its ancient wisdom and practices to a modern knowing of our body, mind heart holistic approach to wellness. His articulation of a scientific approach accompanied by the photographs and illustrations is a true yoga manual for in-depth study and realization.

Later, in early 80s, two students of his wrote a book titled *The Sivananda Companion to YOGA*. Swami Vishnudevananda wrote the foreword. This manual with its beautiful and concise teachings and visuals with specific chapters on various aspects of yoga is one I always recommend in my teacher training. In its simplicity it is a wondrous text for how to live the practical life of yoga. In his foreword, Swami states, "In conclusion, I would like to tell you that yoga is not a theory but a practical way of life." This is so true to my experience!

Ah, now Hollywood meets a female yogi named Indra Devi in the 1950s. Indra Devi's book, *Yoga for Americans*, was also one of my first readings/studies. This paperback book was a mere $2. Its introduction states, "...Indra Devi has brought this ancient art to those who need it most: Americans, victims of a driving, competitive, tension ridden society which suffers from its own superabundance." Wow! The actress, Gloria Swanson, was influential in bringing this powerful healing knowledge through Indra Devi to America. This petite woman, layered in a saffron robe would become an icon of health and wellness in the States and around the world.

When I first opened her book, I recall sitting on a lounge chair in my yard while my children played outdoors with neighborhood friends. I vividly recall reading about the sound of *OM*. After reading about the benefits of calming etc. I practiced sounding a few and to my surprise, immediately felt its deep calming effect. This was the very first time of chanting *OM* for me. I was utterly amazed within the chaos of a backyard filled with young ones' energies, I felt a centered calming that was immediately so soothing and comforting in a healing sort of way.

This book offers a specific six-week course in hatha yoga program for a home practice. She includes basic ten yoga poses, breathing exercises, diets and recipes with a helpful specificity for various ailments such as asthma and arthritis. The book is full of quotes from medical doctors who espouse a more natural way of living and have published books and research. I found this to be so inspiring and prompted me to include more relative research in the hatha yoga aspect of yoga and its many benefits.

Today, of course, there is an abundance of medical research over many years now into the holistic health modalities including yoga. Yoga with its all-encompassing system including spinal movements, breathing techniques, relaxation and meditation processes are being studied with results for healthier hearts, lungs, concentration, injury prevention and healing, mental depression and anxiety, sleep disorders, autoimmune diseases and a plethora of other imbalances. You can find these studies widely viewed on all social media platforms, as well as information on medical websites. Always check with your physician and find a teacher with experience in helping others with the above who has the knowledge and sensitivity to guide you.

*Tomorrow is a fantasy, today is your
reality. Let's do this today!*

Now, with abundant enthusiasm, let's create a space in your home/workplace free of clutter. A clean environment with room to freely move your body, expand your mind and heart will enhance your practice. You may also place some special items that you feel fond of and inspired by in your space. Perhaps a special gift, candles, stones, crystals, incense, pictures of your spiritual inspirations, nature, statues, writings. I have so many beautiful, inspiring works of art and objects mostly gifted to me by teachers and students throughout the fifty years of my journey. Whatever inspires you place in the environment where you begin your practice, sadhana. Let your special place feel to be your unique sacred area to deepen your yoga practice and even a place to pause, to regroup, to return "home" within yourself. It will be a place of refuge, peace and calm. Your evolving light energy will also begin to fill this space and become a beautiful inner and outer environment for inspirations.

A "Yes, You Can!" and "Yes, You Will" space!

Now know you can also practice yoga even before getting out of bed. So let the decorating of a yoga space not distract from your actual practice. Sometimes this can be a distraction for procrastinating. The procrastination and excuses can be crazy. "Do It Now" is a saying from yoga master, Swamiji Sivananda to his students.

Just breathe!

Sacred Heart Sequence

THROUGHOUT MY LIFETIME practicing yoga, I have shared thorough, deep revelations, discoveries through my explorations and my own journey's pathways this lifetime, which facilitates a field of exploring, seeing, discovering, knowing and enriches the felt experience of witnessing a new way of being in body.

Now having said that, one such remarkable movement flow practice surfaced and held my deepest attention one morning. Within a resonant vibration from my Tibetan bell, I entered as if being led, taught by someone in Spirit a simple yet profoundly moving heart-centered movement sequence. The Sacred Heart Sequence birthed into a space and time of now with familiar ancient tones, waves of aquatic life and mountainous reaches throughout eons of earthly and galactical pulsations and rhythms of life. A mutation of species swarmed and swirled through my body. Beneath my arms a supported and guiding presence elevating them toward the space through sky, my heart arched and was the center of all movement, the initiatory point of expression. As

I continued being awed within this wondrous matrix of movements, I began articulating the value as I flowed through and into this direction a pose unfolding and another and yet another, all the time being led from my Heart!

This was during my usual morning sadhana before I ventured out to teach a few yoga classes. My teaching usually is very inspired by my morning practice. This, however, felt very different with importance and inspiration within its sacred sequence. I arrived at the facility with an abundance of enthusiasm and when I began those classes, I shared my morning revolutionary mystical experience with my Sacred Heart leading the way. As I shared the sequence initiating from our Heart, pausing to create a Sacred Heart intention which we see clearly and feel deeply, the classroom filled with curious participants, and we began and the flow of breaths and movements with deep Sacred Intention and a sincere exploration throughout each sequence. The morning this was given to me, I shared what I experienced as the Sacred Heart Sequence from that very day and each day since.

This truly remarkable moment I knew I must share as a simple, yet profoundly powerful yoga practice for anyone, everyone, anywhere! The potential to have the Sacred Heart Sequence become a daily practice of deep living prayer, grace-filled and life-affirming, love flowing and peaceful blessing, which all can incorporate each day, was in and of itself profound! I love that many are practicing it at home! I am touched by stories of participants sharing this practice with others and experiencing this Sacred Heart Sequence as a life-affirming way to center, focus and be present in the realm of one's Sacred Source.

May the simplicity of this Sacred Heart Sequence encourage you to practice as a devotion each day!

Sacred Heart Sequence

Place both palms upon your heart center. The Sacred Heart space is at the center of your chest. Breathe gentle, soft waves throughout your body-mind-heart. Feel the wave motion of each breath cleanse and release busy, chaotic thoughts, calm chaotic emotions, all which tenses and densifies yourself. The process of letting go begins to occur and deepens. Clear your Heart space for new life, new energy to fuel your heart's attributes of love, kindness and compassion.

Settling within your Heart, mind-body-heart aligned, pause to feel and see a sacred intention arise, appear as a gift to yourself for this new day. Take your time, relax within your body, feel layers of muscle and joints soften, let go and quiet the chattering mind and feel the space of your heart unfold with each gentle inhalation. The field of Knowing will be clear of past and future and you will enter the *Present* moment of life and See with a crystal-clear clarity your gift! Your Sacred Intention can be a visual and affirmation presented to you from your higher deeper knowing, your Sacred Source, your soul's journey.

Hold it gently upon your body-mind-heart with each breath, allowing it to take root. Feel it flow through the soles of your feet into Mother Earth as a connective blessing. Feel it stream through tributaries as an energy flow within nerves throughout your body and throughout the spacious landscape of your mind. Nurture it with your attention and breathe life into its form. Throughout this day, in this way, honor this as your gift and treasure it as a blessing from the Sacred realms.

And now we move with a divine inner dance from our Sacred Heart.

Let's explore now with our Sacred Heart Sequence a way of clearing, energizing, rebalancing and experience our Living Prayer Meditation. Rooting our experience within our body. Not leaving our body to pray, meditate but *including body* in a wholistic presence of the Sacred.

Tadasana

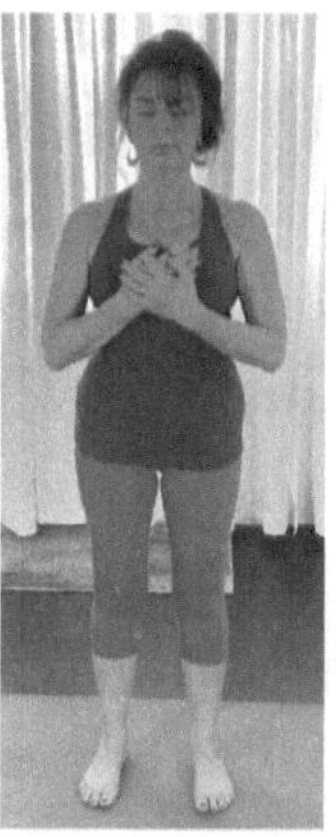

Our Sacred Intention is set/focused we feel our feet supporting as we stand well-balanced upon the earth. We soften our knees, which are usually locked due to being out of our body and sink our roots through the earth's layers. Gently let our hands float away from our heart space and place them beside our thighs. Allow your shoulders to soften, relax, and gently turn your palms just a tad forward. This simple intention. Feel it rooted within you as we continue.

Forward Bend

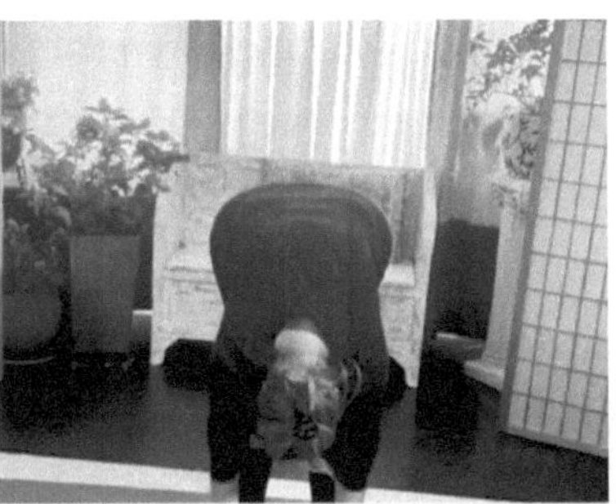

We continue now with our head slowly tilting downward toward our chest, let it hang with your jaw slightly opened and relaxed and let's warm up with simple, slow movement of chin toward right shoulder, take a breath, then return to center and move it toward left shoulder, breathe. Do this simple pendulum-like movement a few times, allowing the neck to loosen and free of tension.

Centered chin with chest, let's do a slow roll downward feeling our spine curl naturally, relaxedly. Bend knees a bit until your fingers touch the earth. Pause and breathe. Acknowledge the Mother Earth supporting you, your homebase in the vast universe, from which you live purposely upon with each breath, with each heartbeat. Send through your hand, a prayer to/for the Earth. It could be an offering of Sacred Intention as well. Let's walk our fingers on the earth, in front of our feet out further without compromising being centered on our feet. Soften our knees a little more, gently pull our thighs back a bit, arch our hearts gently upward, eyes looking up and breathe strength through our hearts. Few breaths with this holding movement then relax with head arms hanging. Repeat if you like.

Staying in this forward bend, let's roll up just enough so our arms, hands are inches above the earth. Then with simple outward circles from our shoulders with arms hanging loosely, invite the electrical current from our central nervous system out into our whole body-mind-heart! This simple movement is a way of inviting and welcoming a healthier electrical current to flow through the tributaries and stream throughout our energy systems. "Welcome! Come out and fill my body with vibrant health and wellness today!" With this simple gesture and exclamation, we participate in our health and wellness rather than waiting for it to happen by chance. We empower ourselves!

And now, with head, neck hanging, relaxed, knees still soft not locked, gently roll up, unfold your spine slowly, use your belly muscles not to contract but to support with the rising up. Returning to Tadasana, placing palms upon our heart take a moment and root, align, balance. Pause to feel the flow of energy released and received from the forward bend.

Arch Angel (Arch your heart—reach and receive!)

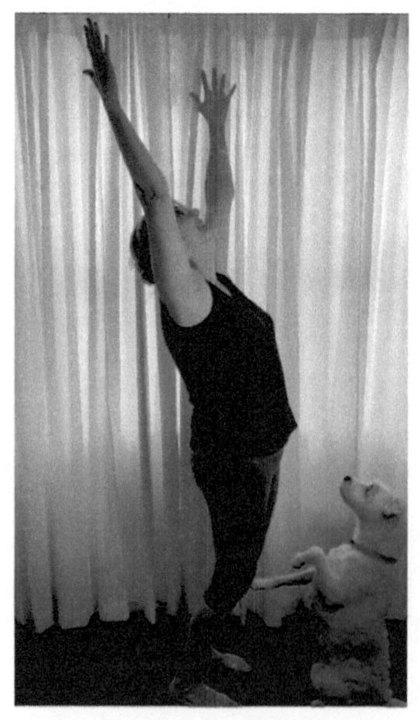

Our palms gently float away from our Heart and upward toward the sky, toward a vast universe of creation some refer to as heaven. Our arms now reach, outstretched for the blessings and gifts from your Sacred Source, whatever, whoever that is for you. From the center of our Heart "Reach and Receive" the fuel, the Prana, lifeforce, you need for this day and feel it being absorbed and flowing freely throughout the tributaries of your body-mind-heart. Reach and Receive the blessings and gifts of a new day, a new beginning. Enthuse your body-mind-heart with this realization, a "Wow, I woke up for a new day!" kind of exciting energy!

Trust with all your heart, you will be given all you need for your day. Greet each new day this way, each morning with deep-felt appreciation and wonder! Feel from the depths of your heart arch toward the Sacred Source and the love, the divine love you receive and are connected with in this movement!

Your breath is the umbilical cord which connects you with all of life, including your Sacred Source! Breathe fully, deeply and energize the Divine within your cells! Radiate with the Light of the Sacred!

Place palms together above your head in a mountain pose for a moment, feel the strength and stability of the Sacred Mountain support and fill your being. Rooting the blessings you just received with this Yoga Mountain pose enables an integration of your gifts from your Sacred Source into your body, layered within the mind and your sacred heart. Palms together, with deep gratitude for this connection with the Sacred, they return to your Sacred Heart space. Place them upon your heart and pause to feel the energy experience of the arch. Sensate the vibrant Prana, lifeforce you received. Feel into the sacred nourishment you received from your Sacred Source this morning. Gratitude!

Lateral

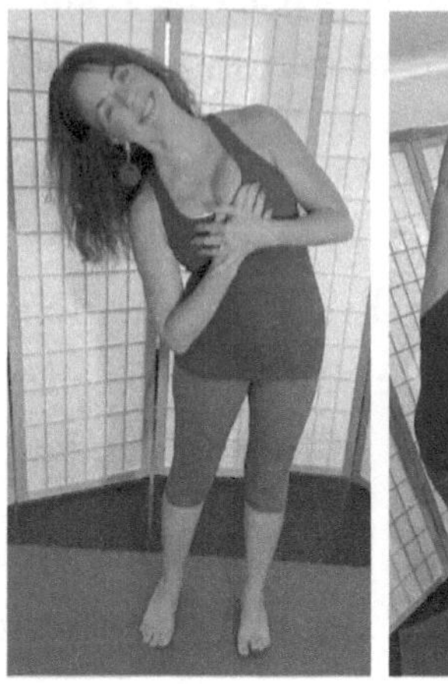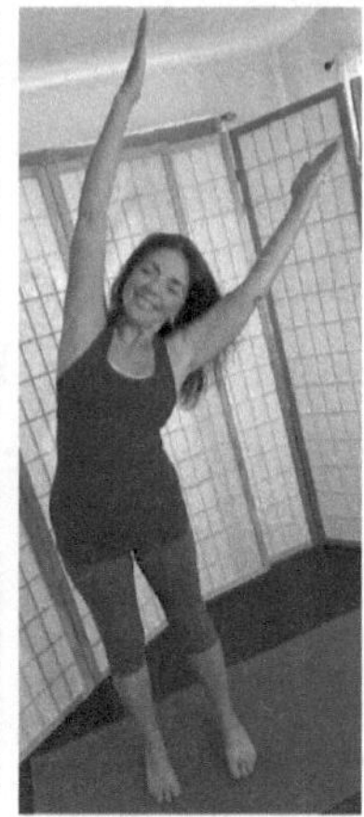

We feel the fullness of the blessings we just received within the depths of our Heart and now allow our wings to unfold gently out from our sides, expanding from within the center of our Heart. Soften the joints while suspending the arms in this T-formation and begin to side bend from your waist to the right, soften the right knee, eye gaze out in front of your heart space, now begin to wave the arms toward the head and back out to the T-formation with a gentle fluidity. Feel the movement initiated and flowing from your Heart out through your angel wings/arms. Graceful, easeful a few moments reach the arms over your head to the right. Pause to breathe into this side stretch of your spine. Sensate the unfolding of your body and feel this lateral stretch of your spine. Return upward with arms in a T-formation, using the side of your abs to lift you, return to Tadasana pose. Repeat, gently returning palms to your heart after flowing to the left side with same, pause with undulating waves of your wings first then placing them in a stretch to the left over/beside your head. Return gently to Tadasana.

Palms upon your heart, sensate the release and receiving of energy from two lateral moves with wingspan left and right. You may even experience yourself naturally waving the body after your wings took flight through the air. Your Heart energy lightens you!

Sacred Spiral

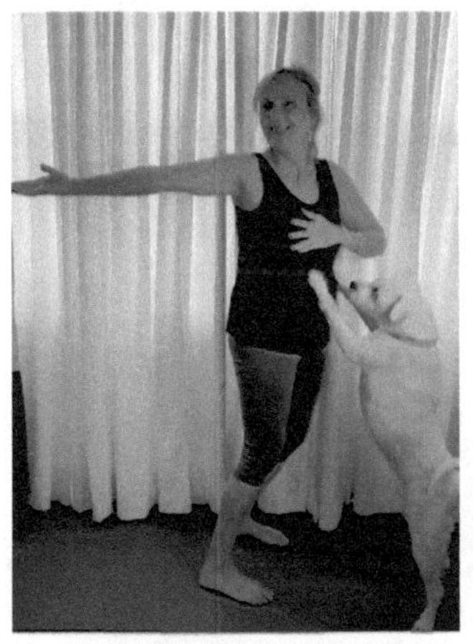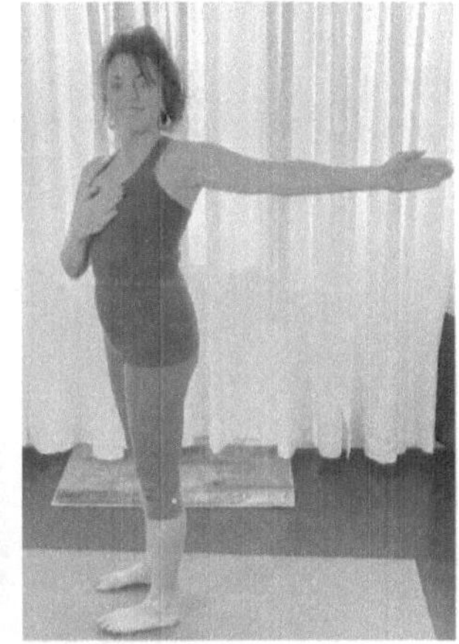

Our palms feeling the quickened pulse and waves of new life Prana, from prior movements, we now unfold our wings once again, outward toward a soft T-formation. I emphasize soft so we are not focused on an outcome of intense stretch/posturing, but rather with soft unfolding of your wings, your whole self into the day being centered from your Sacred Heart.

Our arms outstretched gently, elbows, wrists softened, knees softened, we initiate from our waist a spiral movement, twist to the right, feel the spiral slowly move from our waist upward through the rib cage, shoulders and neck. Look up over your softened palm and breathe life through the center of this sacred spiral. You can add a wave of your arms upwards and out into the T-formation a few times with fluidity, if you like, then return floating forward.

Continue floating with wings opened to the left now. Feel the air currents supporting beneath your wings/arms, look up over your palm, breathe through the center of the spiral, wave your arms upward and back into T-formation a few times, then gently float forward. Feel the buoyancy of floating and being supported by waves of air!

We return our palms upon our Heart and pause to sensate the release of energy and lifeforce from the spirals. We feel the pulse of new life, the wave motion of prana moving from our Heart throughout our whole body, layered within our mind, heart and spirit!

Sacred Heart Sequence Completion

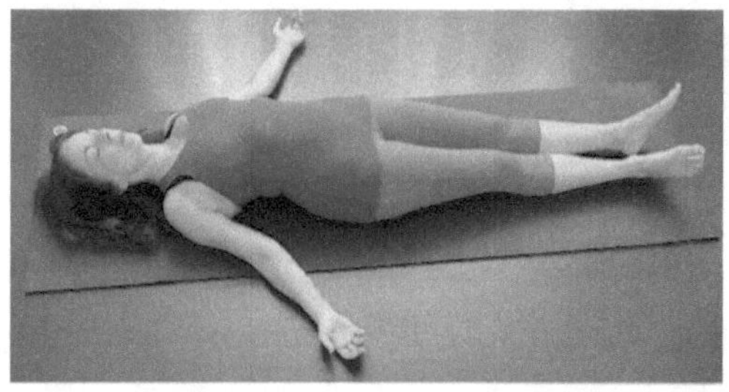

Pause, resting palms upon your Heart, and with eyes closed "see" the energy field circled and surrounding you. Feel its vibration pulsating all around you with Love, Kindness and Compassion. Now a vibrant healthful energy you created is expanding within this biofield of YOU! You created this with your deeper focus and intention, with connecting through the depths of your Heart's field of Love, with the gestures of your wings, and the spinal movements, unleashed the potent electrical healing lifeforce within your field. Your auric energy field now a clear, light, radiant and loving

Presence. Love's Presence is pulsating from your Sacred Heart throughout your field!

Warmly welcome this sacred Presence within your deepest heart of heart's each day! Warmly enthusiastically "reach and receive" the blessings of a new day!

Warmly and devotionally begin your day with this simple yet very profound yogic way to pray, meditate and be engaged, aware and full of wonder with a Sacred Heart Sequence!

You can improvise and include a prayer you are fond of, or a wish, or affirmation with each sequence. Make it your own! Feel the Divine Presence supporting and streaming throughout you.

I truly feel this Sacred Heart sequence will bring Peace, Love and Joy throughout the world! With its simplicity and profound magical and mystical connection threading a universal tapestry of Sacred Love from our Sacred Creator Source, it can and will be so!

Simple Yoga Sequence

THE FOLLOWING SEQUENCE and variations can be practiced any time of day, anywhere you have a little space to move. Let's appreciate how yoga is not as complex and challenging as some would have you believe by their acrobatic, pretzel-like positions, complex athletic sequences, hanging from straps, backpacks filled with equipment and the cool look of yoga attire. Be comfortable and explore with a simplicity!

Here we will focus on its health benefits from a simple practice, which takes a few moments of your day. You will feel such wonderful shifts in your energy and feel a calmness right away! You will be encouraged to give yourself this simple dynamic practice as a special gift to yourself each day!

We will move with simple six directions of linear movement of your spine. We will next add the breath flow with the movements. Thirdly, we will add a deeper sensating, somatic awareness, of these movements. We will move from *learning* the movements in a cognitive way to *entering* these movements with our full open attention and curiosity. Be curious about the new fields of possibilities and perceptions that will unfold before your very own eyes! How exciting!

Here, we need a little more space for more movement as we place our yoga mat on floor for a lying-down practice. Let's begin with a simple warming up, loosening up and breathing up our bodies!

Practice slowly and gently, with loving kindness for your body, whole self. This attitude is everything in a yoga practice or any practice actually.

Let's begin by lying down upon your yoga mat. And we shall pause to sensate our body, what we bring to our practice, where we feel tight, constricted or soft and pliable.

Breathe!

Bend your knees, place feet apart on your mat, arms resting beside you for this moment and sensate each breath. Follow the breath throughout the body where you feel it. Your back wall moves with the waves, neck and shoulders feel a micromovement with breath. Unlock your jaw. Can you sensate breath affecting movement upon your face, roof of your mouth, around the cranial vault, your palms, feet, hip, pelvis, legs, arms?

Subtle waves create movement throughout your body. Let your breath gradually increase now and continue feeling the unfolding from within, the Prana begin to flow throughout you. Such a privilege to breathe on our own, isn't it?

Roll

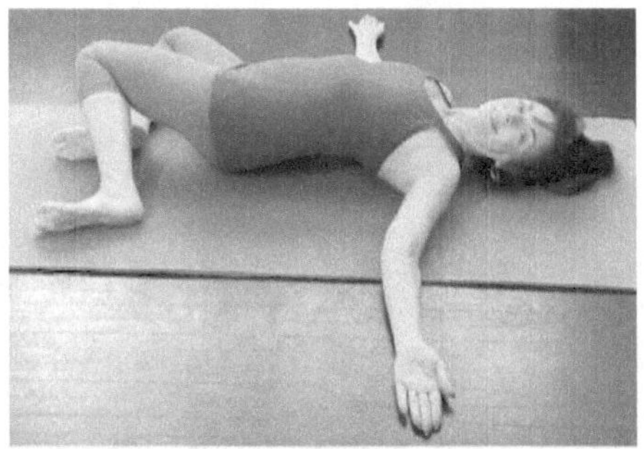

Gently begin to roll your head left to right. After a few slow rolls here then invite your legs to engage in the rolling, opposite of your head. This is such a sweet way to initiate a yoga practice on your mat. Eventually come to center with your head and knees and now gently roll/press your lower back curve toward the mat. Release with a delicious sigh. Repeat a few times.

Now let's open this further. Feet apart on mat, turn them and legs down and over to right side near the floor and your head/neck opposite turning left. Try not to scoot the feet but simply turn them over where they are on your mat, apart. Pause in this simple spiral and take three deep breaths, sighing all the way down your waist into your left hip area. Return slowly to center and repeat opposite sides. So now your feet and legs turn over and downward left toward floor, head rolls right. Pause, breathe with a sigh and slowly return to center. Feel the release and let it go.

Leg Extensions

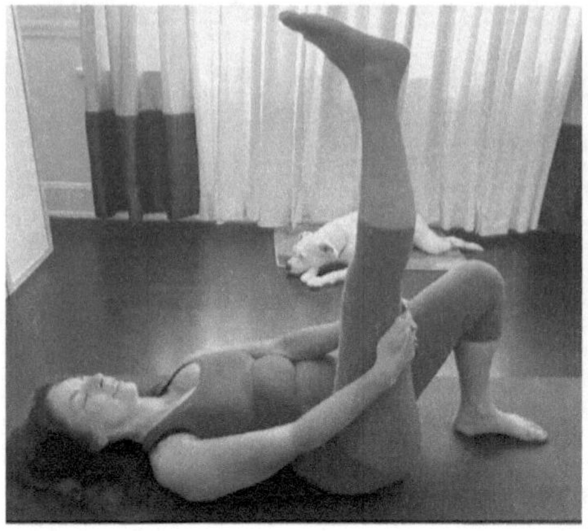 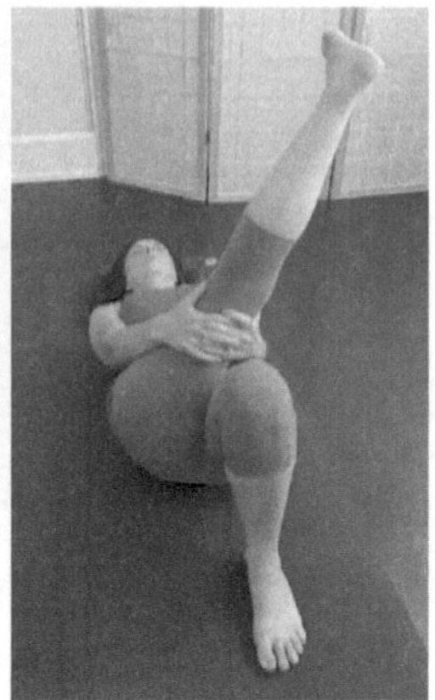

Bend the right knee toward your chest, relax the foot and lower leg, and rock the leg side to side, then circle from your hip. Unfold the leg upward with palms intertwined behind the mid-thigh for support while you stretch. Gently push the thigh forward to your palms to lengthen without locking the knee. Now with this stretch, cross the leg over left and pause here. Relax the knee then stretch it out a few times slowly. Palms still supporting behind your thigh. Return to center after a few circles of foot and pause to flex the foot up and down.

Place your right hand on inside of knee to hold and left arm slide out to left in a T-formation. Move the right leg halfway to the right, holding with hand, soften and stretch out knee, then resist your palm when returning leg to center. Do this a few times, then release your hand and lower while extending leg forward right above mat, flex foot few times, turn foot out to right and skim above floor your leg toward your right hand which is in a T-formation. Hover here above the floor, soften and stretch knee, then slowly return upward, bend the knee and place foot on mat. Pause and feel the difference, right/left leg. Place your palms atop hips and feel the difference! Amazing! The right one will feel more nestled within the joint, the left a bit protruded. Now to balance with other, left leg repeating the moves above mentioned. Start by supporting your leg with hands, cross over stretch, soften, stretch and return to center. Left hand now holds inner knee for movement/stretch to left. Resist hand returning leg to center. Release hand and leg now moves down and forward, pause above mat flexing foot a few times, turn it out to left and move slowly toward your left hand.

Hover above the floor, soften, stretch knee and slowly lift up to center. Bend knee, place foot on mat, palms atop hip bones. YES! Feel both balanced and nestled into socket. So simple to take good care and balance yourself!

Knee to Chest

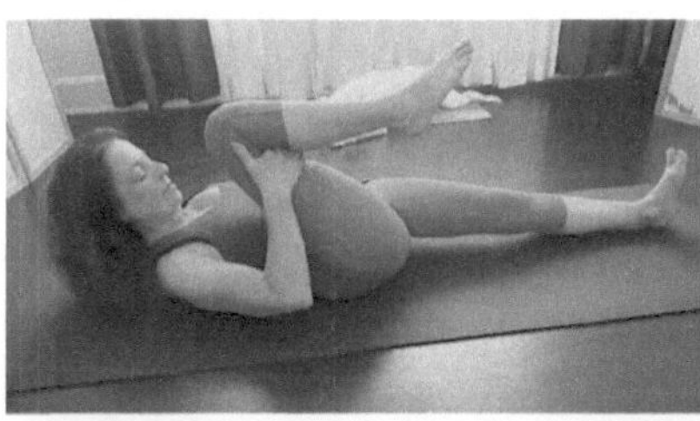
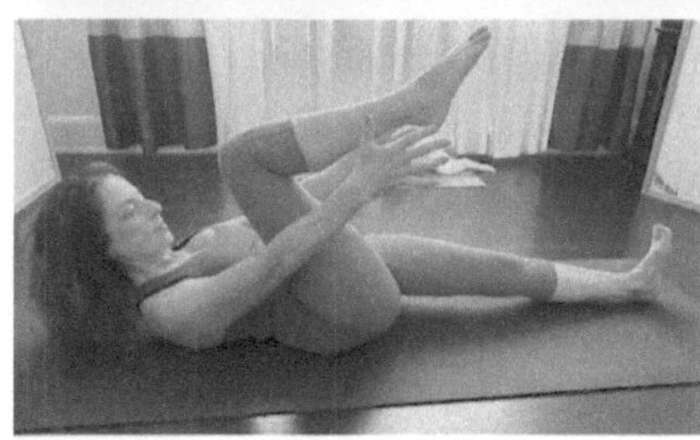
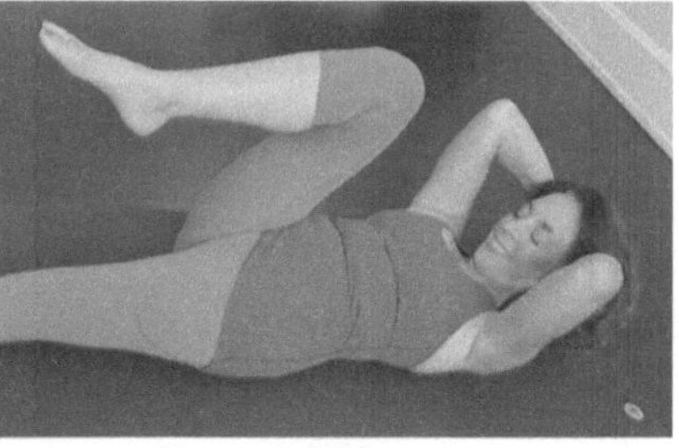

Bend right knee toward chest and place interlaced hands behind thigh. Inhale and on the exhale, slowly curl your head up to the inner knee. Check to see your lower leg is not bowed inward but is aligned with hip. Hold and breathe. Support back of head with your palms now, elbows in toward face. Lower the head an inch above mat and totally support weight of head into your palms. Pause and breathe elongating your exhalation all way to tailbone, pelvic area. Few breaths, curl head to inner knee using your arm support on head.

Few breaths, then lower head gently to mat. Lower leg out in front also. Pause, feel, let go. Repeat with left leg and include the head in palms also for a subtle cranial sacral release movement.

Our hands are placed behind thigh rather than upon knee to enable a movement with fascia sheath from lower back, leg and buttocks. Also gives knee a gentler bend.

Pause and you can now do the same forehead to knee using both legs. Hands placed behind both thighs, head curled toward inner knees. Knees are bit apart, lower legs aligned with hips. You can hold this pose extending your arms forward also for an added deepening of strength in abs.

Support your head if needed when you have a neck strain. Place palms together support back of head with elbows in toward face.

Relax afterward with knees bent feet apart on mat. Pause and feel a release in lower back.

Spinal Twist

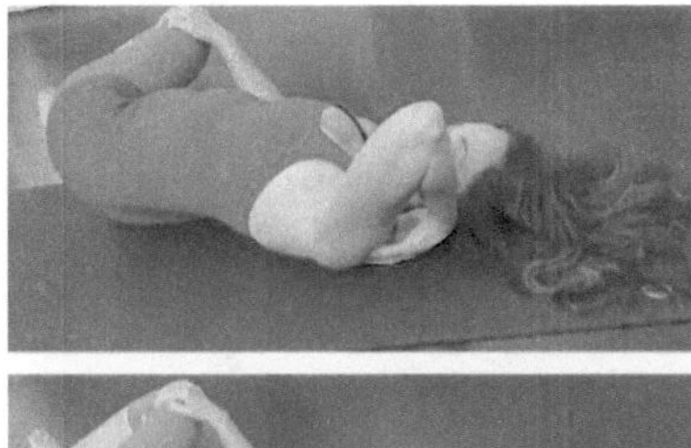
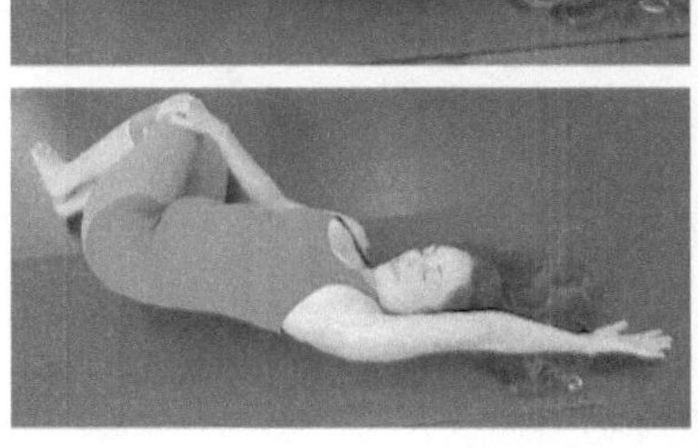
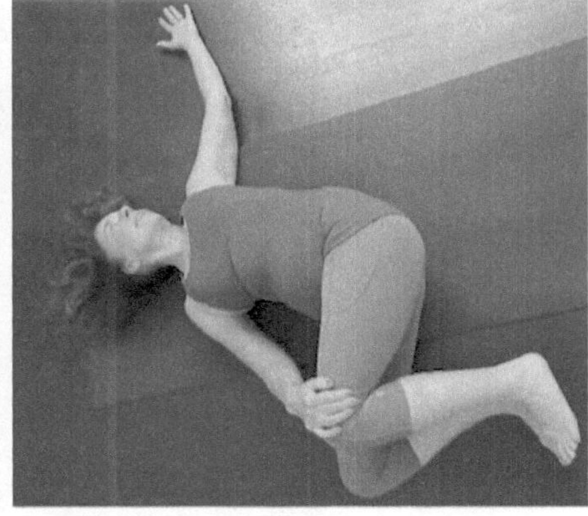

Both knees to chest, arms in T-formation with palms turned upward. This position of your palms enables shoulders to roll back toward mat. Be aware of shoulders in this movement keeping them as best you can upon your yoga mat. Now let's move both knees halfway to right and rock halfway to left. Do this simple rocking motion slowly with legs bit apart. On third move to right, place them on floor near your right elbow. Place your right palm on side of left thigh for added stretch encouragement. Roll your head gently left looking toward your left palm. Pause and breathe deep sighs throughout the spiral. Feel your exhalation reach down to your hip.

Center your head, bend left elbow and place fingertips on your shoulder. Make few outward circles with your elbow to loosen shoulder joint. Now lower elbow back toward head and unfold gently your left arm in a delicious stretch. This expands the stretch with deep breaths. Hold for few breaths, return gently arm in T-position. Slowly return knees to chest and repeat on other side now. Pause in a hold of each position and breathe sighs down to your hip. Feel how breath moves and the sound of sighing waves through tissue and creates deeper releases. It finds the tight, misaligned spaces and creates healthy change.

Slant Board/Bridge

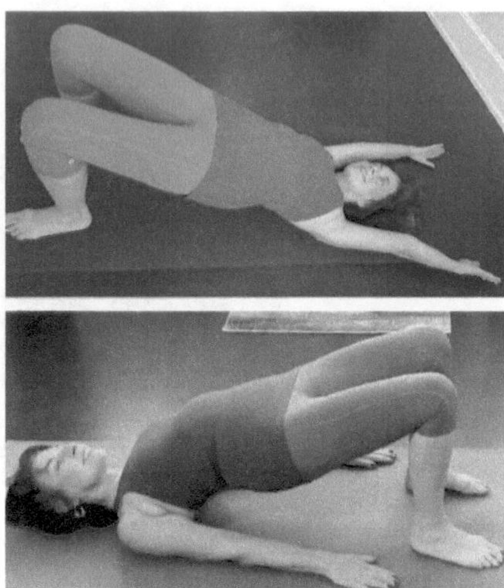

Knees are bent, feet on mat apart aligned with hips. Feel the whole foot upon your mat. Feel into the center of each foot for balance. This is where you will initiate the lift in a moment. Also, bring arms close to your sides. First, turn palms up, enabling shoulders to roll toward mat, then palms down. Let's take a moment and feel the centeredness of both feet, rooted to the earth. And feel the fatty part of shoulder muscles upon your mat. Take a few breaths, then on your next exhalation, press feet into your mat to begin slowly elevating your back up off floor and landing upon large muscles of your upper back. NOT on your vertebrae!

Feel the weight still centered on your feet, knees aligned with hips and begin the delicious sighing. Feel your belly receiving the sound and lengthening. Pause here for a few breaths then slowly, evenly (not wiggling back and forth), begin your descent upon your mat.

Pause and feel the relaxation throughout your body including your abdomen. There are also some variations which can be included. For instance, once up in this pose, you can reach your arms behind shoulders, stretching them, breathing, then slowly lower your back while stretching your arms. This is such a wonderful stretch of your back all the way down to tailbone. Rest afterward, always pause and feel a release. Feel a difference and energy flow.

Child Pose

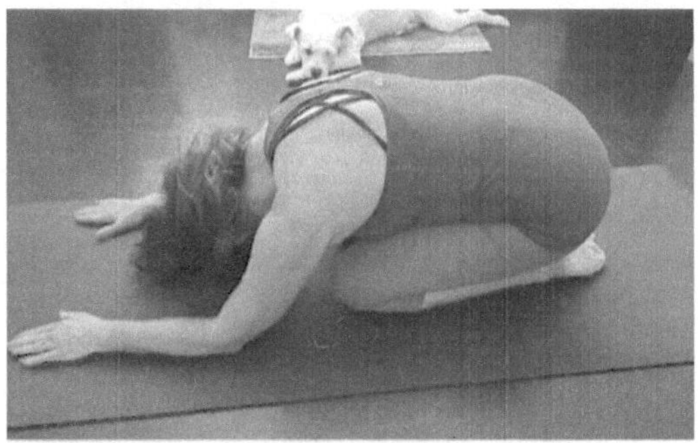

Now roll over, sit upon your heels, place forehead on mat or upon your folded arms, prop, and relax your arms beside you. Feel your shoulders sloping toward mat. Feel the waves of your breath undulate throughout your back, your neck, your head. Feel a rhythm within these waves which is deeply massaging you, soothing you and in this pose feel you are intimately returning home to yourself. Dr. Fulford told us this pose creates the dynamic flow for cranial sacral process. He highly recommended it each day for practice.

All the busyness of a day melts away, as you feel a deep welcoming home within yourself! Linger here a little longer and feel the folding inward to and with and for yourself.

Cat Pose

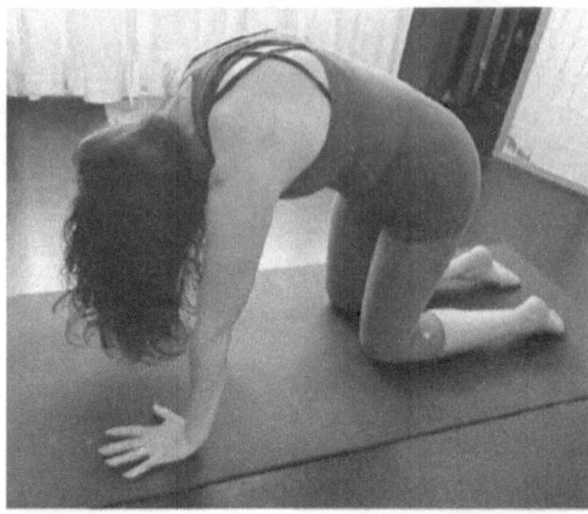

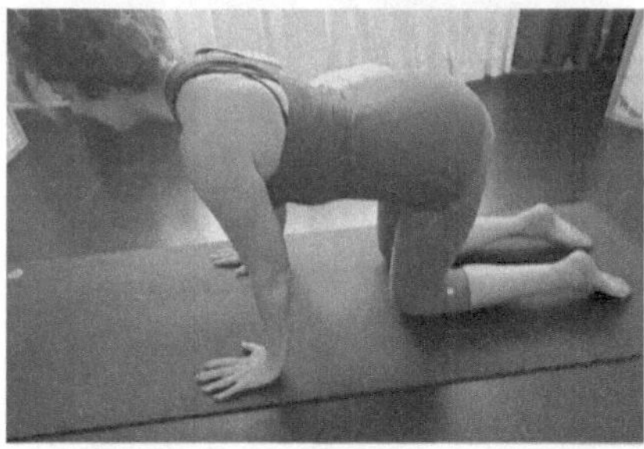

Begin in a table position, wrists beneath shoulder, knees beneath hips and feel a slight move of arms inward toward fatty part of thumb. This helps with eliminating pressure and outward rotation of wrists. Pause and breathe and feel your foundation.

Begin moving your shoulder blades upward arching toward ceiling and feel the extension from palms, wrist through arms to shoulder blades. Let your head, neck hang relaxed. Breathe a few breaths to loosen tightness from within. Breath waves will undulate through layers of muscle and tissue bringing more malleability to this chronically tense area of your body, upper back, shoulders and neck.

Unfold slowly moving chest slightly forward in a position in between wrists. Eyes look up, head tilts upward slightly, elbows bend back (not outward) slightly and pause, feel the strength of upper arms and back. The lower back is in a neutral stance and not exaggerated curve. Breathe a few breaths, then gently return to your child pose, rest arms and breathe.

Repeat the above a few times with detailed cues for positioning of your foundation.

Variations:

a. With first position rounded shoulder blades toward ceiling, draw your r. knee near forehead. Unfold into second position and extend your r. leg behind you, toes on floor and tilt hip toward mat. Now slowly lift leg in air using your thigh, buttock muscles. Hold and slide your l. arm forward and lift slowly upward. Soften this lift in your arm to enable the arch to initiate from your Heart. Smile, enjoy balance, strength and flexibility! Repeat this using opposite leg and arm. Rest in your delicious Child Pose and absorb the effects.

b. Practice again bringing r. knee to forehead as detailed above. Now bring the leg to the side of your hip and place leg on floor with an extension. Instep of foot turned onto floor. Slowly slide the knee inward toward your hip and slide back out into an extension a couple of times. Pause, reach with heel and slowly lift leg even with hip, breathe while holding, feel the deep strengthening on outer thigh! Return leg slowly behind you, stretch it upward with extension and return knee on mat beneath your hip. Follow with the left leg now and after rest a moment in your Child Pose.

Dog Pose

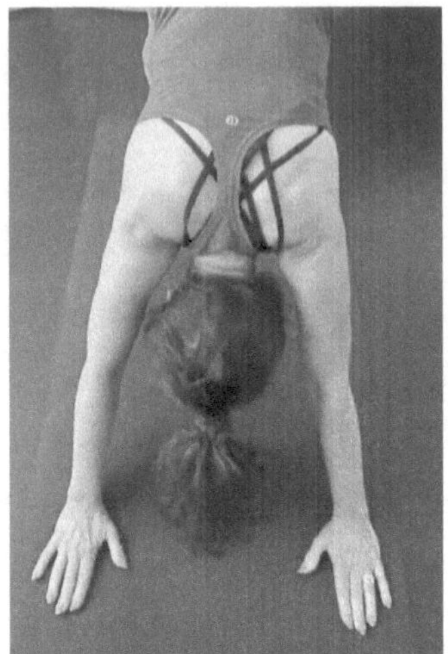

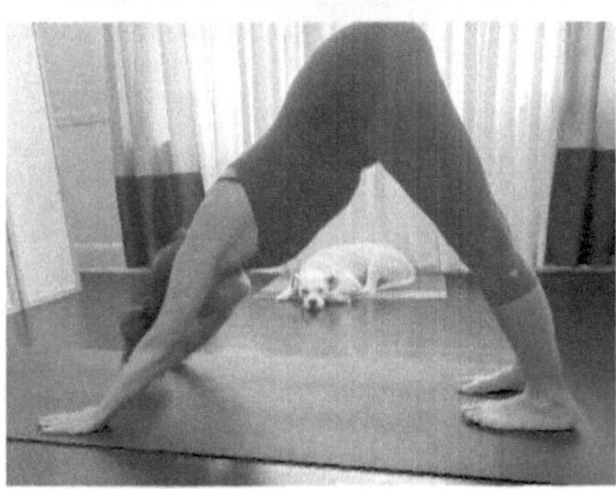

Assume your table position foundation. Focus first on your hand placement. Palms pointing forward, middle finger straight ahead. Now initiate arm rotation slightly from shoulder blades down arm to fatty part webbing of your thumb. This practice is important to avoid collapsing of elbows and misalignment of upper body while in Dog Pose. It is part of the beautiful symmetry of the whole body during this asana practice. We have your hands properly placed with arms rolling inward toward your thumbs. Lift both knees same time slowly and look down at your feet. They should be hip width apart. Soften your knees and move your chest down and back toward them. Pull your thighs gently back toward wall behind you with soft knees. Hold and feel the lengthening of your spine, the strength of arms support, the tailbone moving away and upward. You breathe, you feel and let tensions dissolve from your body.

Descend with both knees at same time lowering upon your mat. This keeps healthy symmetry intact and avoids any SI joint irritations.

I see so many flexing, releasing one side then the other, but you are misaligning with this way of stretching in Dog Pose. Let your breath wave throughout your body while holding and you will reach even deeper areas to release and let the dynamic stretch occur!

Variation:

a. Enter Dog Pose with cues from above, hold and breathe. Slide r. leg back, toes on mat, tilt hip downward and then lift leg up behind you. Again, check hip and keep facing it toward your mat to avoid twisting lower back. Hold, breathe and move center of chest back a bit more if you can. Keep those lovely arms rolling in toward thumbs. Lower leg back down upon mat gently, feet aligned on your mat and now move your l. leg, slide it back, tilt hip downward then lift with an extension. When complete lower knees simultaneously upon mat entering your Child Pose. Pause and allow your body to absorb the beneficial results.

Sitting Poses

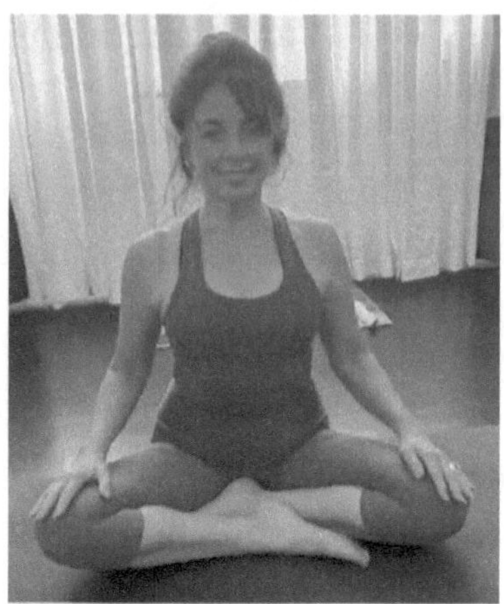

Remember, your six spinal moves include a forward bend, arch upward, lateral r. & l., spiral r. & l. and your breathing and your gentle wave motions. So, let's begin in a sitting position upon the floor. These movements can also be done in chair or even sitting on the edge of your bed. Depending on your degree of comfort there are so many cues to enable your comfort and maximum enjoyment. Let us begin, cross-legged and sitting your buttock upon edge of taut blanket or pillow. On the edge enables knees to relax as well as hips. Begin by placing fingertips on your knees, pressing slightly to lift your waist and find those sitz bones for proper alignment. A nice deep sigh to your butt will enable a release and balanced rootedness for sitting experience throughout your poses.

Sitting Forward Bend

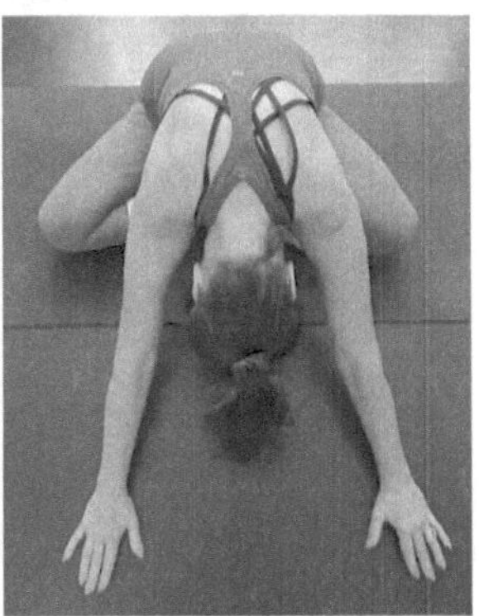

Now, breathe to center and upon your exhalation bend from your waist forward. Try not to scoot off your sitz bones. Hang forward a few breaths. Slowly ascend with neck, head last to come up. Use your abs more in the lift. Pause and absorb with a smile. We went down now we move in opposite upward into an arch. This also can be variated with legs extended. Be sure not to lock your knees.

Sitting Arch

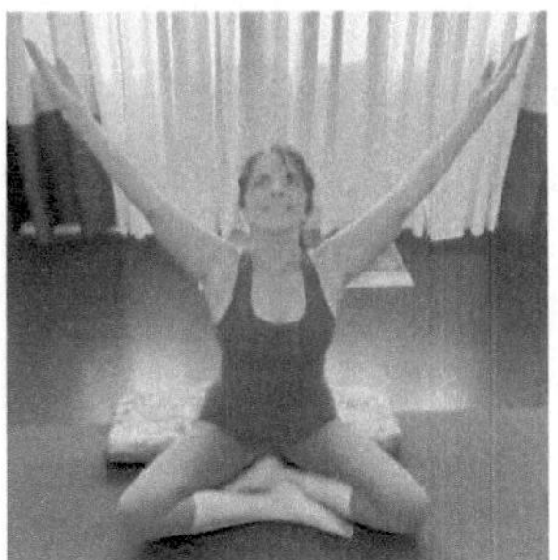

Balanced on sit bones, inhale, exhale let your arms float upward toward the stars, sun and moon. Lift from your heart center and not by bending neck; eyes looking upward and reach for the blessings of this beautiful day! Palms spread open, heart lifting into an arch of a new day and receiving the gifts of new life! Feel each deep inhalation unfolding you to receive all that you can this moment.

Arches are so exhilarating and expansive! After a few breaths, slowly lower your arms and rest them upon your lap. Pause and feel the lightness of your body, mind, heart and spirit!

Sitting Lateral

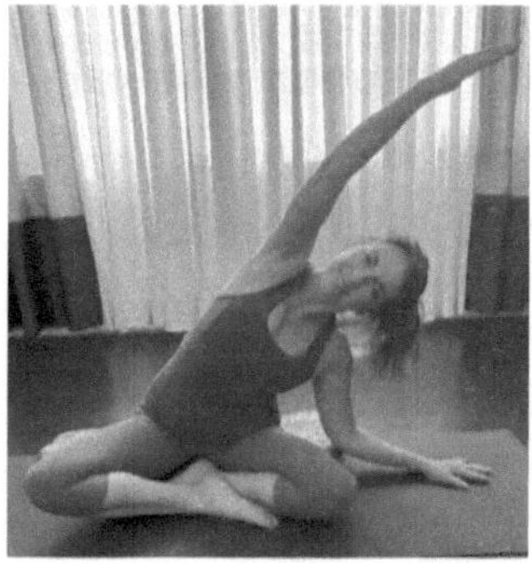

Sitting on sitz bones, palms upon your heart, begin to move your wings/arms outward to a T-position aligned with your shoulders. Feel this extension initiate from your Heart. Inhale then exhale the move side bending to your right from your waist. Place your right palm onto your mat and aligned with hip. (This avoids a forward collapse of pose) Let's wave the left arm though the softness of air and space then gently stretch it over the side of your head. Hold and breathe.

You can also be sure to gently press your left sitz bone to mat and be amazed how this simple movement opens the stretch! When coming up, extend left arm in T-position and the right as well, lift from your waist, not your neck leading! Use those abs, my friend!

Continue after a pause to sensate difference, right/left side, to move now to the left side. Same as above, arms/wings in a T-position, bend from your waist left, place palm on mat aligned with hip. Wave your right arm gently, feel the softness of air through your fingertips! Stretch the right arm over your head, hold pose and breathe throughout the body. Return gently, arms in "T" use your waist to lift to center. Pause and enjoy the benefits!

Variation:

When in your side stretch pose, you can also lift the arm from mat and place both arms beside head, reaching out in the stretch for a deeper strengthening of abs. You can also interlace fingers and turn your palms outward. All is so delicious. Take your time to pause and enjoy as you continue to explore.

Sitting Spiral Twist

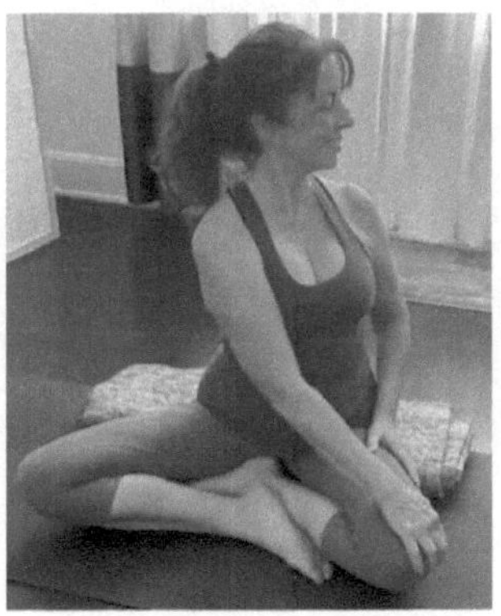

I love spirals and the sense of when you wring out excess water from a washcloth, so here you are wringing out deep tensions with a tremendous flow of circulation afterward streaming throughout our whole body. Pause and feel your balance sitting. Initiate the movement with hands on side of right thigh and press gently to lift your waist and heart. Begin turning to the right from lower waist and working your way up from rib cage to neck. Eyes wide opened look up over your palm. Most people look down and under and neck is compressing. Avoid this by simply maintaining a horizontal plane for your eyes to follow.

Return slowly, unwinding gently and repeat other side. Let your shoulders relax in the spiral and afterward when sensating the immediate response when you release.

Standing

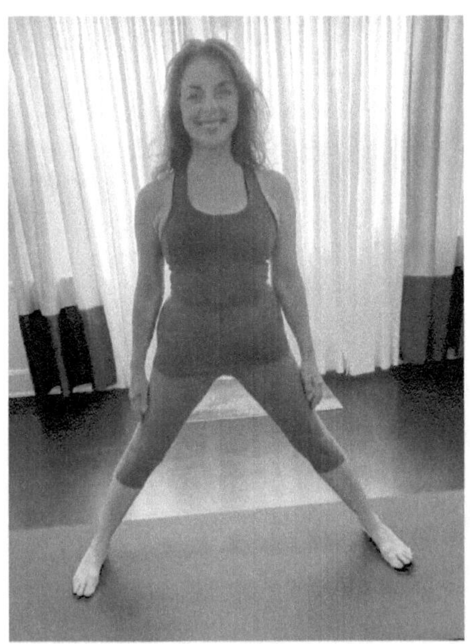

Standing with feet slightly apart (8" or so) and feel center of your soles upon your mat. Feel you are well-balanced on your feet. Your hands rest beside your thighs with a slight turn of palms forward. Now soften your knee muscles without bending the knee joints. Pause here and breathe. Rooting into the earth you will feel a natural symmetry where bones align, and you center with breath waves.

This will feel so awkward perhaps at first, because we are always out of balance standing. We tend to lean forward on balls of feet and lock knee joints or lean back on heels with pelvic tilts that misalign our whole skeletal system. Sink downward into center of your heels more.

Practice this each day when in line somewhere like a store etc. and you will begin to feel a natural centering and balancing begin to occur soon. Now that's exciting!

Variation:

Stance

Widen your stance about 3'. Feel being centered on both feet and not turning ankles out or in. Be aware of not locking your knees. With this stance you can proceed to repeat the above six spinal moves. Also, you can proceed with the following. Take your time and feel into your foundation a balance and rootedness. Be aware of alignment. Note if you are leaning forward because you are looking at floor in front of you. Keep eyes out in front gazing in the horizontal plane in front of you. Now you are ready to explore deeper moves, deeper meaning, deeper joy! How exciting!

Trikonasana/Triangle

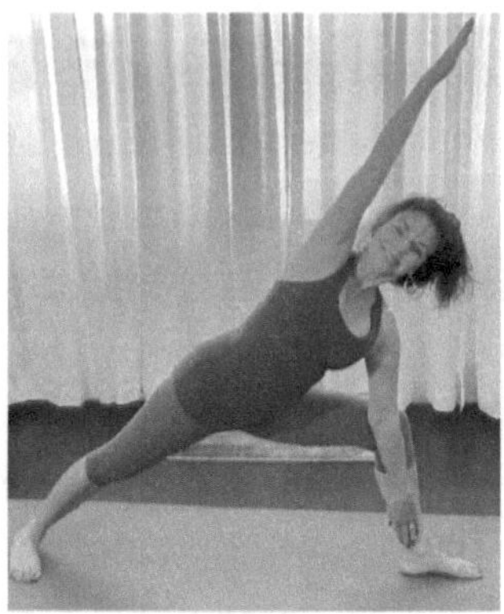

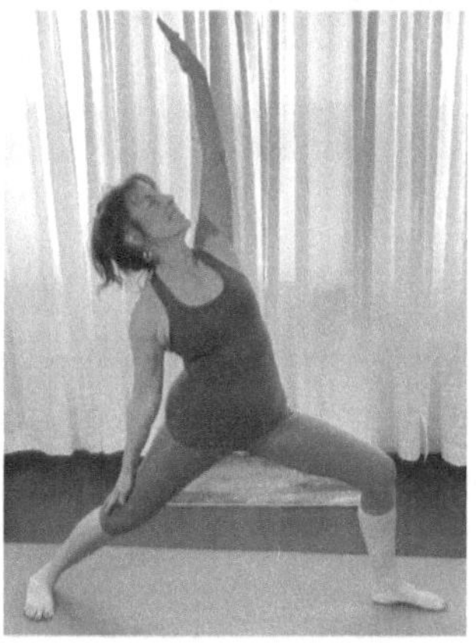

Pause, feel feet centered on soles, soften knee muscles allowing a deeper rooting. Inhale, exhale, and extend arms in T-position and turn/pivot on heel, right foot to the right. Inhale, lengthen torso and stay centered, exhale and bend rt. knee as much as you can to a right angle, hip-knee-ankle aligned. Inhale, exhale bend waist over and down to right and place rt. hand on inside of lower leg between ankle and knee. Avoid going to floor. Hold this pose, lengthen your torso, feel your left foot rooted not turning in ankle, breathe and come with waist leading the lift. Be aware of not using your neck to lead into or out of poses. This I see often.

Continue on left side with the above Triangle pose. Add on the arm in air extended over the head, lengthen ribs, waist with rooted feet. Check your ribcage from rolling forward.

Spiral/Spinal Twist

Arms in "T", soften knee muscles and turn slowly to rt. from waist, ribs, neck, head. Pause and breathe, feel breath's waves move through the center of the spiral unfolding and releasing deep tensions. Now while holding this pose lift both arms upward beside head, reaching for the sky. Return forward and repeat on left side.

Forward Bend/Chair

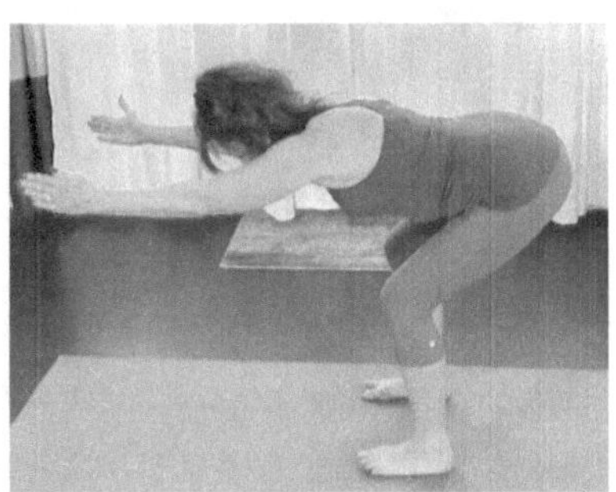

Arms lift up beside head, reach away from waist, and begin bending forward while keeping arms in this stretch. Just go to halfway, torso parallel with floor. Breathe while reaching forward, be centered and rooted on feet, soften knees and gently feel behind thighs a stretch to wall behind you. Hold for few breaths, then fold down toward your mat. Pause and relax. Roll up slowly and pause to feel the release.

Warrior

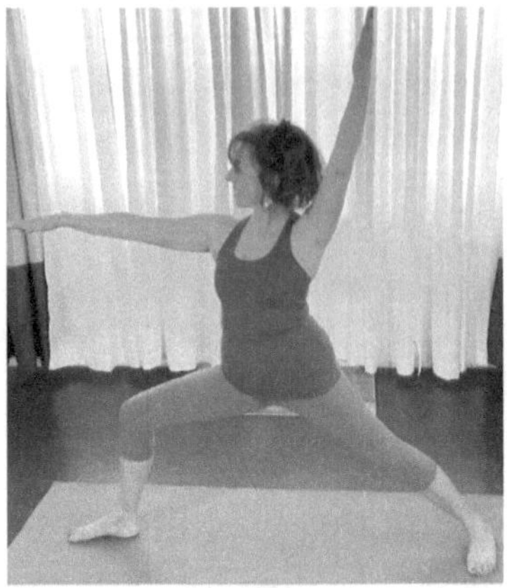

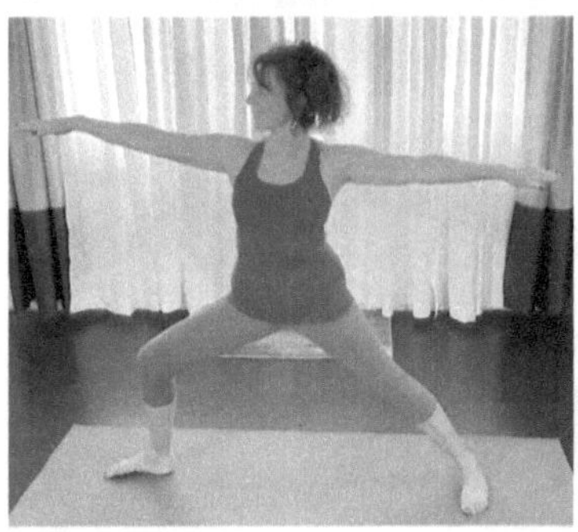

Peaceful Sacred Heart Warrior! – Arms in "T" feel centered in your power and strength. Slowly pivot/turn on heel your rt. foot to right. Look over your rt. hand. Inhale and lengthen then exhale slowly bend rt. knee near to a right angle as you can. Left arm lifts up behind your head to complete the warrior stance. Well rooted feel the left hand as your warrior's antenna reaching to receive the electrical current of Prana, it flows through your Heart and out through your right arm hand into your field and life.

Now take a few breaths and feel your whole self absorb and take on the stance of the peaceful warrior. The heart of the peaceful warrior for justice and love!

Tree

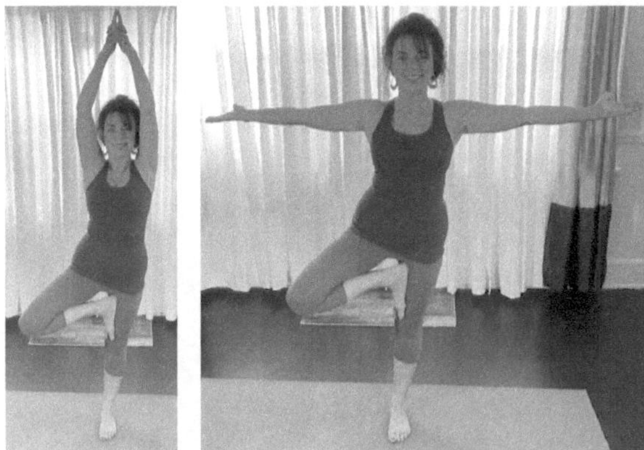

Begin standing in your balance Tadasana and pause to feel the soft flow of your breath and the rooting of your feet. Initiate movement of arms out in T-formation, pause here and feel the center of your belly supporting in your lift as well as legs. Now let your right foot float slowly upward, placing outer ankle on top of left thigh. Arms float up and hands come together in prayer position.

Feel the deep rooting of your tree into the earth's energy, feel the arms and hands as the branches reaching out into space and feel the center of the torso a strong and resilient trunk.

You can use a chair beside you and lightly place fingertip on it without leaning into it though, Practice for being well balanced in your body. Calm and centered too.

Partner Yoga

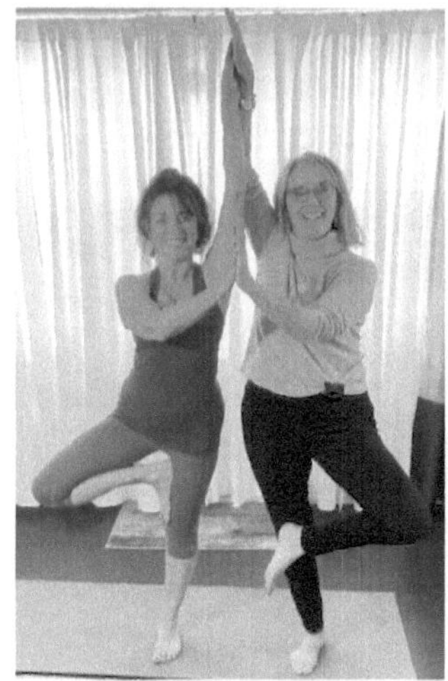

It is fun to also support for balance and extra stretching with a partner, as you see my friend Vickie and I in the tree pose. Be sure both of you are well-balanced in your foundation and have fun with it! Other poses such as forward bends and arches can be experienced with a partner, too.

Hatha Yoga Breathing Techniques

BREATHE! We tend to hold our breath or breathe very shallowly even when practicing yoga. This is one of the reasons I highly recommend a private session now and then so I can see and point this out and help with various breathing sessions a deep release of breath throughout your body. Breathe gently when pausing and sensating. Breathe spaciously when in and holding a pose. This will bring a deep fluidity and resilience to your body-mind-heart.

Relaxation

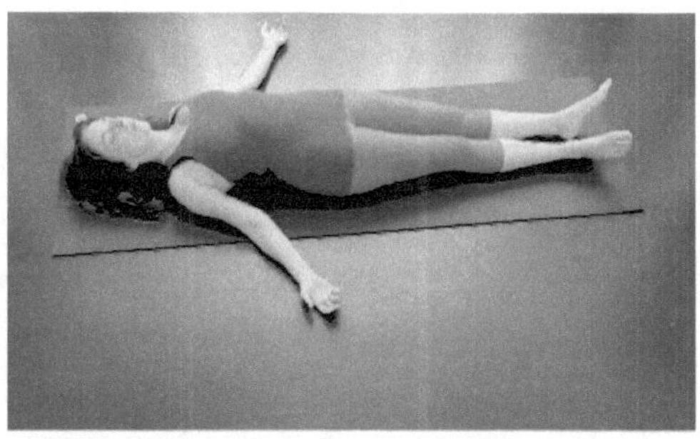

I always tell beginners this pose of Sarvasana is actually I feel one of the most difficult to master. I share as I did earlier in my book, my response in the first time I entered this in Lilias's class. I was stunned by the constant chatter that filled my mind and affected my body with anxiety.

Let's begin lying down comfortably on your mat. You can support beneath your neck or knees with a small roll of a towel, blanket or a yoga soft prop.

Begin by sensating the breath at the tip of your nose. Note what your body feels like this moment. Scan from feet upward and note any sensations of tightness, tensions, misalignments. If your mind wanders off, and it will from time to time, do not be frustrated just return to feel the breath.

Feel deeply through layers letting go and responding to your gentle kind attention and release into a luxurious healing relaxation. Take your time, repeat if you like. Unlock your jaw, let your lips part a bit and feel the structure of your face soften. Your eyes soften and space in between your eyebrows soften too. All around your head and scalp feel breath soft flow and lightness.

Linger in the presence of your breath's soft waves and feel the calming peace flow through you. Of course you can practice this yoga relaxation anywhere, anytime in any position. However, this pose will deepen and enhance the experience.

Enjoy and take a few moments after to roll over on your side, curl up and create an affirmation of wellness for yourself. See and feel it vividly and deeply. Come up slowly, use your arm strength with head hanging forward to easily sit up.

How do you feel? Practice each day a few moments.

Deep Rhythmical Breath

Be comfortable, let your shoulders soften and jaw relax. Slowly inhale through your nose for a count of ¾. Hold the breath comfortably for same count. Then slowly through the nose release the breath for a double count of 8. Repeat, slowly deeply inhaling and comfortably holding breath, relax shoulders, soften forehead, eyes, and exhale slowly a long exhalation.

This breath is excellent for increasing your lung capacity to breathe and for slowing you down.

Connected Breath

Inhale through nose a deep spacious breath and sigh with the vowel sounding *aaaaaahhhhhh* through your mouth. Inhale right away through nose, not mouth, and sigh out a long *aaaaahhhh-hhh*. Eventually you will be charged with energy and a release of tension because of the sound vibrations.

I tell my students when teaching this breath, what happens

when you enter an elevator. Everyone is immediately quiet and holding their breath unconsciously. So, I inhale and sound out a deep sigh. The effect is contagious, and you will see others breathing more deeply. Try this sometime. Of course, you will also receive a few looks but hey, you all are breathing!

There are myriad breathing techniques like alternate nostril, *kapalbhati* (fast-pace respiratory exercise), intense abdominal movement, cleansing breaths, etc. I am keeping this simple purposely as I stated before. The two above breaths balance each other vibrationally and are amazing with immediate results.

This simple sequence initiated from your Sacred Heart will unfold many layers of energetic currents to nourish you in so many ways, friend. Enjoy a simple yoga practice and its many benefits starting today!

Meditation for All

BEYOND RELIGIOUS AND philosophical belief systems, meditation can be an attribute for a deeper experience of your own path. Meditation itself is not beholden to any one particular area or region of the world and certainly not owned by any religion or philosophy. It is a universal practice.

Meditation can enhance your body-mind-heart-spirit with a direct physical, mental, emotional and yes, even spiritual well-being experience. The simplicity is amazing when one desires to explore meditation for the first time or if you are well adept for eons in a meditation practice.

Let's keep it simple. Let's do this together! YES, YOU CAN.

I want you to read through each practice such as the first "Breath" then put the book down and practice for a few minutes. Note how you feel before and after. Pause and really take it in. You can even create a journal for notes in the back of this book to see your journcy progress! Take advantage of these pages and journal a few lines. As I mentioned at the beginning of my yoga journey in 1973, Lilias's book, *Lilias, Yoga and You*, there was a one blank page section for notetaking. I did so and still enjoy reading my ten-week progress when I began in 1973!

Let's begin your journey this moment, this day!

Preparation: Sitting either against a wall, upon a cushion, or lying down. Sitting helps you to stay more aware/awake in the process. Sit upon your sitz bones on edge of a firm cushion as this helps your knees to relax forward. Against a wall, be sure to scoot your tailbone against baseboard and shoulder blades touching wall. Preferably your head touching it also. Sitting in a chair again, be sure your tailbone is all way to back of chair, shoulder blades comfortable on chair back, feet resting in alignment on the floor.

Of course, you could lie down as well, but one tends to fall asleep. If you have insomnia, this is good practice to enter sleep and experience a deep restful sleep.

Sitting or lying down, you are now ready to explore meditation. The health benefits are numerous, and we will share them at end of this chapter. Ready? Let's do this!

Again, read through each practice one at a time and put book down immediately practice. Give yourself few hatha yoga moves to loosen a bit the body, then sit properly and begin the practice. Allow for a few minutes at least and please do not be discouraged when you see/hear your thoughts flying all over the place. This meditation practice will clear and calm the mind, soothe emotions, and bring a healthful balance to your body-mind-heart. It also has the capability of enhancing your spiritual experience.

Enjoy the journey, my dear friend. Let me know how your practice is going and how it is enhancing your health and wellbeing!

Practice #1 - *Breath* – More often we hold our breath throughout the day, and when we do breathe it is so shallow barely noticeable. Layers of tension within the body occur with this shallow breathing patterning we have and don't realize. Mind is rampant with constant half sentences. Let's see if we can create an inner environment of peaceful calm with our breath. I am certain you can/will my friend!

    a.   ***Breath Sensation*** – At the tip of your nose sensate the touch of breath's softness and lightness. Feel it's coolness upon inhaling and warmth exhaling. Your mind will wander off here and there just return your attention and feel the breath there at the tip of your nose. Feel your face's structure begin to soften, your eyes, jaw, shoulders and neck and eventually down through your belly, back, legs and feet. The softness of the breath's gentle whisper is softening tensions held within your body and quieting the busy, chaotic mind so it may rest.

Practice a few moments upon awakening in morning and before entering sleep in evening. Let yourself increase the moments of this practice gradually.

Use it throughout each day when you feel tense, frightened, overwhelmed, chaotic. You will immediately return to your center of your power and be in control over anxieties rather than them wreaking havoc in you!

b. ***Whisper Breath*** – Inhale through nose, then gently, slightly open jaw and audibly exhale a whisper from back of throat longer exhalation. Close mouth and inhale through nose again repeating the exhaled whisper breath with mouth softly opened. It is a vowel sound like, AAAHHHH which is whispered. Feel your heart soften, midback, shoulders too. This relieves tension anxiety held within and surrounding chest area.

Let your inhalation be slow and easeful. Same for your long, exhaled whisper sound. When you have completed few rounds, pause and feel the space of deep quiet and calm. Just linger in this quiet comforting inner space. Let it deepen. Let the benefits be absorbed and felt. This will encourage more moments with this breath.

Practice #2 – *Sound* – First let's practice. Then afterward let's discuss this mantra AUM/OM and all of its qualities and possibilities. It is an ancient sound practiced for centuries in temples, in various religious circles and yoga classes and individually to create a deep, centered calm and a higher vibration. We know all throughout the universe including you and I are resonating with a vibration frequency. Even modern medicine is using the sound vibrations to diagnose and for healing.

This ancient practice of AUM is a simple way to create a higher frequency which helps our body to heal, our mind and hearts to align with all that is one with the Sacred Creation. The small stuff which distracts us day in and out fades away, and clarity and purpose and courage with love elevates ourselves in deeper ways. Let's dive into this sound of letting go and healing. Yes, you can!

a. ***Mantra AUM*** – Let's begin with a deep, easeful inhalation. Exhale with the sound of AAAAAAAUUUUMMMMM for entirety of your exhalation. Close mouth, through nose inhale slowly and deeply again and exhale the universal sound of AAAAAUUUUMMMMM. After a few practices it will become a natural sound of healing and comfort for you. Feel this simple mantra reverberate on roof of mouth, throat and how it softens your heart. Its higher frequency gently awakens all your energy centers for optimum health and vibrant living! Practice this sounding for a few moments, as long as comfortable then relax into a silence and feel the movement of silence deepen. The Aum will resonate long after you stop sounding.

Aum Shanti Aum Shanti Aum Shanti…Aum Peace, Aum Peace, Aum Peace be with you, my friend!

b. ***Solfeggio Frequencies***-Sound Therapeutics is gaining momentum. Uses of various frequencies with tuning forks are used to assist in relieving stress, muscular tensions, headaches, injury healing, trauma and mental imbalances as well as overall tuning for a vibrant health field. It is being used for cancer and other diseases not limited to any organ or gland, the entire biofield of oneself is receptive to healing sound waves. You are comprised of 70% water and water is a conduit for sound waves. The healing resonance can be remarkable.

Nowadays you can access a personal treatment with healing therapeutics (I provide in private sessions and retreats) or there are numerous YouTube and apps and recordings which provide the

Hertz frequencies. If on your own, simply find a recording, practice few yoga movements and rest in Sarvasana relaxation pose. Feel the breath waves calm you, and just pause and absorb the sound waves. Linger after also and make a note of how you felt before and after the healing experience.

Practice #3-*Movement Meditation* – Here we enter into a deep Somatic Movement dive. Instead of "doing" six spinal asanas/poses, we now explore this field of our whole self, body-mind-heart with a freedom of allowing movement to be initiated from deeply within. We allow the wisdom of our body to express itself freely, subtly without our willing or doing the moves. Unpredictability is the key here.

We set this up as a meditation by creating a space, sitting or lying down. Relax the body, few deep breaths and feel a letting go. You can have inspiring ambient music playing to inspire or simply use the Whisper Breath or both as I sometimes do. Simply deepen and expand your moment of pausing and allow a micro current/wave to be felt perhaps through a finger, toe, shoulder, jaw. It is slow as it emerges from deeply within as an organic authentic expression of this miraculous body. Simply, sensate without needing to name or identify, just allow movement to express itself freely. Ride its wave observing.

There is no right or wrong. This is a deep exploration and expression of the innate wisdom and profound healing capability of yourself. Let the movement be free of judgment and feel into its layered depth. It could be a small ripple through your hand that emulates the undulation of seagrass beneath the sea. It could feel to stiffen, tighten then release. There are myriad expressions of movement just waiting to be released! Movement may naturally, spontaneously emerge anywhere in the body. Just go with the flow as a witness and feel as a participant. Not deliberately directing, but allow it to unfold naturally, and from a new way to sensate such movement. Being the witness rather than doing the movement. This facilitates so many benefits throughout your life! Feel breath gently initiate a subtle wave from somewhere within the body. Let movement express the delicate complexities and unfold its myriad of possibilities in your realm of knowing!

For instance, I may begin to feel my little right finger initiate a spontaneous movement and while noticing and focused with feeling this my left hip may undulate within its socket, or my jaw may feel a release. Just relax and let movement surface from the depth of knowing and creative genius which is innate within you!

I taught and shared this experience in my meditation classes, in retreat settings. I taught a class with this meditation and entitled it Body Play! Let the Whisper Breath initiate a movement, support your movement exploration too. Let your body inner play with movement while you deeply sensate and notice and after a while, are in awe of these organic expressions. Be patient. This takes time to really enter but oh so worth the time and effort!

When you are ready to emerge from this depth of moving meditative experience, just lie there and pause. Relax and eventually breathe more deeply, move fingers, toes and roll over on your side, curl up for a few moments before sitting up.

Without judgment, perhaps write about your experience. In workshops, retreats after group experiences with this movement meditation with micro currents, we also nonverbally will draw our experience. The experience is dreamlike, and our expressions may be beyond words with more abstract expressions. All is good and beneficial. What rhythms are felt, softness felt, energy tingles felt and any difference in how you feel within your body.

Each of these simple Meditation practices have benefits which are lasting. You are well worth being with this deeply a few moments each day! We spend many hours accumulating stress and anxiety why not give yourself a few moments to simply and deeply let it all go! Clear your inner space, quiet and calm the rhythm of your life. You will have abundant more energy and vitality along the journey, my friend. The above ways of entering meditation are simple and can promote profound depth on your journey. Feel Meditation as a devotional practice for your wellbeing.

Spiritually, you can interject a focus of your Sacred Source during any of the above practices. I was told years ago (in 70s) that prayer is a way of **talking** to God. Usually expressing what we need, want in our lives when we pray. Meditation is **listening** for God's response. It is a practice of deepening our ability of being in the deep sacred silence to hear God's word to us. If you are involved in a prayer group, include Meditation as a practice to listen also. Enter the Sacred Silence of your Sacred Heart! Enlighten your whole being! Om Shanti… Peace be with you, my friend.

Just breathe!

Return to Wholeness: Somatic Dives

PHYSICS HAS ALWAYS fascinated me with an attraction to the underlying principles and possibilities with life. *Principles and possibilities* may be a title for another book regarding this pulsing need to explore and know, which I have always felt. Yoga was and still is so inspiring for a number of reasons and one major reason is the ability to enter with a somatic exploration. Linear meets wave and motion becomes m'ocean!

Continuum movement provided a context for exploring beneath the surface and a diving board to jump off and into this realm of new possibilities within a yoga practice. A whole new world of enthusiastic exploring burst open its doors for me and continues to this day. Yoga practice can be a rote set of linear movements sequenced for various reasons such as a particular area of the body needing healing or feeling especially stiff in the morning.

Is your yoga practice a rote set of same asanas you "do" while your mind is elsewhere? Are you landing and stretching in the same spot each time, each practice? Are you entering a practice as a regimented discipline? These are just a few cues to get you to ponder just exactly why, how you practice Yoga and what benefits are you continuing to receive? Be very specific with your answering and you might also want to write down these inquiring thoughts and expand your consciousness with a bit more attention. Just breathe and dive in!

Physics, both mechanical and quantum, have a unique field of knowing viscerally within a somatic yoga adventure. The buzz words nowadays are "deep dives", "embody", to name a few but this real experience is beyond all those noun frameworks of entering. I find in this recent culture of yoga and movement marketing such an unsatisfying and sometimes boring rendition of the actual miraculous experience of sensating a field within yourself that is absolutely untouched, untraveled territory. With a somatic movement inquiry added to your yoga practice, you enter the mystery as a curious explorer and observer. The articulation of this remarkable experience is challenging at best, and sometimes not even needed. Often, we habitually need to place explanatory feedback immediately and minimize the depth and field of possibilities. Allowing a lingering in the pool for deeper knowing to arise with a depth of seeing and sensating is always more remarkable and revealing.

Yoga asanas and breathing is a fundamental useful linear-fashioned sadhana, which can be a diving board to jump off/into the deep mystery of creation, swim through tributaries flowing with currents both watery and electrical, a consciousness unfolding into your mirror to see, feel, and be amazed by. Simple spinal moves accompanied by subtle and spacious breath waves are an initiatory entry into a quantum field of mystery and miraculous wonder of the healing possibilities!

The mechanical linear movements of the spine can be a means to meet the undulating spacious fields of fluid resonance. This meeting can gift us with greater potential for healings of past concreted images, fearful perceptions which have us stuck in the goo of a bare and boring existence. It can unfold and reveal a tapestry so wondrous and connected with all of life including a starry stream of galactical awakening. We can meet with kindness our limitations mostly self-imposed and heartfelt compassion and "reach to receive" the effervescence life is made of, the fluid resonance of love. Love in all its miraculous, wondrous eros and holiness and feel union with the beloved, which may perhaps be love in and of itself. Hence, be loved! Just Breathe!

Invite a new yoga with a somatic movement engagement, not a prescribed image or roadmap, but one of deep exploring without any directive. It is the deep primordial pause I refer to often when I teach, where we meet the unknown and enter its territory of unpredictability with the eyes, ears, touch of an ancient explorer having the realm of possibilities open to travel throughout time and space and feel so enriched by the interconnectedness with all of life, earthly and extraterrestrial. This, my dear friend, in my humble opinion, is true essence of yoga, the union with Love in all its fecundity and fluidity.

When I was first introduced with deeper dives into Continuum with Susan Harper and Emilie Conrad, I was struggling how to continue teaching and practicing yoga because I was so thrilled and bursting open with this new way of feeling movement and new life. Yoga seemed to be fading away from my system as I entered this new experience. Both Susan and Emilie inquired about that with me and especially Susan encouraged me not to abandon yoga, but sense how could I bridge, merge the two. Perhaps this was my pioneering quest to take on.

It was not easy at first. It seemed yoga was "this" and Continuum was "that". It was like going to a gym and lifting weights and hopping on one machine after the other and trying to compare that with a yoga experience on my mat as merging. It took a while as I maneuvered through the yoga and Continuum as two separate practices to finally feel the presence of being and exploring within my yoga practice too. I realized the mechanical linear poses of yoga, when explored with an openness of discovery, I could enter the quantum fields with Continuum simultaneously.

I began noticing how I articulated this blend in the early 1990s, with an apparent new way to language yoga. I felt it peel away layers of instructions, rules, to reach the depth of me as a teacher of a new way to be more deeply engaged, more spacious in my field of perception and participation. Seeing how that would broaden the field of awareness possibilities and healing possibilities where I also was a student and learning from my participants in each class was so freeing in many ways.

Body Play

Body Play was movement exploration, which began with a yoga warm-up then we invited with music, sound and silence to explore taking our body out to play. The emergence of freedom to feel into be it a subtle tiny movement, to large gestures, slithering on the floor in serpentine undulations, whatever it all was held in a comfortable cocoon of respect and permission. Each participant feeling into their own realm of inquiry and riding those waves.

Word was getting around the town and the class was filling up. Was it creative dance, I would be asked. Well, it's the unfolding of our Inner Dance, I would say. Ahhh, Inner Dance then became the title for workshops or presentations I gave at various educational settings such as the Midwest Music Therapy Assoc., or a group in a university, or a day workshop and weekends around the country.

The response was remarkable especially during the dives into micromovement of Continuum origins. The limitations of our everyday normal activities are so limiting for the experience of a vast array of oceans through m'ocean, which is always there, always available and awaiting our arrival. Oh, we can come up with many excuses with time, busyness, family, work, responsibilities to avoid this deeper inquiry. Once you take the dive into those realms within your matrix of connections, fluid resonance embraces your attention and swirls you into a deep inner dance of life. It remains with you forever. This is the remarkable experience. Once you have entered and touched the depth of layers, swim in the tributaries of the holy waters of creation, you are impressed with the touch of the Beloved. Words cannot describe. It is your birthright. For me, it is the manifestation of the Lord's Prayer line, "thy will be done on earth as it is in heaven!"

What? Movement can surface this experience? It is not "doing" movement; it is feeling the invitation to dive into the creative waters which support, flow, create, dissolve into this being of YOU. Riding the waves floating, swimming ashore to new landscapes of a living pulsating, spiraling, undulation presence that feels to fill every fiber of your being with a rich nourishment that sustains you forever. It is a meditation which moves, which is all-inclusive, all knowing, all loving.

Toes in the Water

Let's explore a gentle entering and playfully splish-splash in the creative waters for a moment. Playfully being the key word in this engagement.

Sitting or lying down no matter, just allow yourself to be comfortable in a quiet space for a few moments. Scan the body, loosen tightness with some movement, wave a bit side to side if sitting. Lying down your knees can be bent, feet on floor and rock the knees side to side.

Pause and feel the breath a few moments at the tip of your nose. This is a simple way to feel breath. Let your jaw relax open and feel the inner buoyancy of breath waves through your belly, your back, your hands feeling the subtle waves of softness from breath. Layer your attention by feeling these moves.

Add a sound of a gentle, deep sigh and feel where the exhalation moves tissue, joint, a tailbone or shoulder blades. Maybe a fingertip is noticed with a sensation and begins to freely move. Simply feel. From a deeper interior space feel subtle waves surface and retreat. Feel into the initiation aspect. Feel into the dissolving spaciousness.

There is no right/wrong. Just be in this moment as an adventurous explorer, initiate soft, deep sigh and pause to let it dive into a depth of YOU. As though you were floating in a pool, allow yourself to feel your body supported and floating upon breath waves. Breath waves carrying you into a deep mystery.

A response will eventually occur, be patient, be willing to give yourself time. After all, the amount of time you pile on excuses, busyness all layers and concretizes the body is much greater than this moment. You are now reaching into your creation waters, the holy spirit which awaits your return, your arrival to the waters of consciousness which is your birthright. Float with breath carrying you.

Free yourself of bondage of norms and elicit the beauty and wonder which lies within you! Oh, yes, it does, my friend! You are a shining star in this galaxy!

Just observe and allow movement to be freed up from within. Your mind will chatter, just pause and feel your breath. Thoughts will gradually disappear into this ocean of waves. Deep twists of past traumas may unwind and wash away into the ocean. Feel subtle pulses, undulations emerge and just ride those waves. Let judging or predictability fade away, feel the sensation carry you into new territory. Give time for this exploration, free a space from distractions and let the dive deepen.

You surface when you are ready. You will know and feel this too. Let the experience linger and feel its effects without judging or again, having to concretize it with definitions. All in due time this will unfold. For now, enjoy!

Pause and be grateful for giving yourself this deeper exploration and experience. Relaxation will have a whole new meaning and depth for you now. And you will be able to reach within and return to the depths whenever you need and desire.

My yoga practice has never been the same. The mechanical and quantum have merged, and it is with such gratitude to those who took the time to mentor me along the way. These inner landscapes sometimes I rest upon and engage in conversations with my teachers. Even though they are no longer here, their counsel and encouragement live on within these waters of wonder.

When I teach somatic movement and blend the yoga or teach yoga and blend the somatic movement it is a mystical, magical movement moment which bring tears to my eyes now as I write. How blessed I am to have met these icons let alone receive their generosity of time, sharing in such unselfish ways the broadening horizons of a higher vibration, a higher consciousness, a higher Love.

Thank goodness for their realized writings and the foresight to record moments of teachings that I can access as I did yesterday and often when I feel a desire to connect with them. Their brilliance is beyond my imagination, and I continue to learn, to articulate, to be inspired. One such recording, Emilie is interviewing another somatic genius, Don, and she mentions when she taught in Ohio at a Jesuit center. I light up as this was right down the street from me back then. Yes, I attended this weekend! I recall when Emilie asked me to enter the circle with her to demo a point she wanted to make while answering an attendee's question.

She spoke of our ongoing relationship and the trust and honor we have as she answered an inquiry from a movement teacher about working with people one on one. I will not forget lying there listening to her words, soft touch of her hand on mine and as I turned to look, her smile and eyes which stream from a depth of being and knowing which kinesthetically is transferred. I will forever viscerally remember that moment of teaching, literally hands on. After the day was over, and she was leaving I took her to the airport. Before that as we had a bit of time, we stopped by my house which was nearby the retreat center. I was then teaching Continuum in my home and wanted her to see the particular area and bless it with her presence. This blessing was my silent request, and I was so honored to share this space with her.

I mentioned in a previous chapter, the deep inner work with Emilie and Susan and that it was Jean who first introduced me to this phenomenal journey. Ten-day retreats, weekends in New York, San Francisco, Susan coming to Cincinnati a few times to teach with her unique, sensual way of being in the intelligence of these creative waters all were and still so influential in my approach and my own journey.

My dear friend reading this, let yourself explore within this vast and miraculous wonder of creation which is YOU! Simply "reach and receive" the new day each morning, all the blessings and connections. I hope our paths cross someday and we can share together with a somatic yoga experience.

Reach and Receive!

Intricacies of joints, tissue, fluids, glands, organs, breath, electrical and chemical currents, sound waves, thought waves, emotions, energy fields, pulsations, light. *Tat Tvam Asi!* That thou art!

Your body is an electrifying field with constant flux and deep undercurrents of movement which is a beautiful matrix of dances with complex choreography throughout the universe. And maybe beyond?

You are the substance of stardust and oceanic spiral shells with a cortex of genius computer engineering all functioning together and lighting up our galaxy.

You are a poem awaiting expression, a canvas longing for colors of your deepest nature, a dance yet to be choreographed, this is your innate constant unfulfilled longing which is never filled with "things" surrounding you. It is your very purpose to sparkle and shine your most vibrant light and life!

Each of us a part of an amazing intertwined, interconnected INNER DANCE with amazing purpose and possibilities for the entire universe in its evolution! Sound grand? Well, it is!

So, what function may a somatic yoga practice have within this miraculous structure of atoms, cells, tissues connecting, tissues with issues, tissue absorptions of times past, present and future? What on earth did these ancient yogis and contemporary somatic deep-sea divers of somatic realms of exploration into the body-mind-heart-spirit discover? What mysteries were revealed and allow to spontaneously unfold into a vast system of practical knowledge for maintaining a vibrant health and growth for this galactical presence of our body?

You are the one we are waiting for! You are one of the facets of the gem of creation we await to witness in your depth, your unfolding, your unique contribution to this beauty of life on earth, your wisdom, your sacred gifts we await with abundant enthusiasm. Your discoveries on your unique path.

Yes, you can! Let's do this together.

For over fifty years, Diana Devi has pioneered healing therapeutic pathways for yoga and somatic movement practice. She is a popular teacher, mentor, and lifestyle coach who shares her healing insights with a unique approach to body-mind-heart-spirit wholeness. Diana's "Yes, you can!" attitude inspires all whom she serves.